EVERYBODY WANTS TO GO TO HEAVEN
BUT NOBODY WANTS TO DIE

ALSO BY AMY GUTMANN

The Spirit of Compromise:
Why Governing Demands It and Campaigning Undermines It
(WITH DENNIS F. THOMPSON)

Why Deliberative Democracy?
(WITH DENNIS F. THOMPSON)

Identity in Democracy

Color Conscious: The Political Morality of Race
(WITH KWAME ANTHONY APPIAH)

Democracy and Disagreement
(WITH DENNIS F. THOMPSON)

Democratic Education

Liberal Equality

ALSO BY JONATHAN D. MORENO

Impromptu Man:
J. L. Moreno and the Origins of Psychodrama,
Encounter Culture, and the Social Network

Mind Wars:
Brain Science and the Military in the 21st Century

The Body Politic:
The Battle Over Science in America

Undue Risk:
Secret State Experiments on Humans

Deciding Together:
Bioethics and Moral Consensus

Ethics in Clinical Practice
(WITH JUDITH C. ARONHEIM AND CONNIE ZUCKERMAN)

Discourse in the Social Sciences:
Strategies for Translating Models of Mental Illness
(WITH BARRY GLASSNER)

EVERYBODY WANTS TO GO TO HEAVEN BUT NOBODY WANTS TO DIE

Bioethics and the Transformation of Health Care in America

AMY GUTMANN
AND
JONATHAN D. MORENO

LIVERIGHT PUBLISHING CORPORATION

A DIVISION OF W. W. NORTON & COMPANY

Independent Publishers Since 1923

NEW YORK   LONDON

For information about permission to reproduce selections from this book,
write to Permissions, Liveright Publishing Corporation, a division of
W. W. Norton & Company, Inc., 500 Fifth Avenue, New York, NY 10110

For information about special discounts for bulk purchases, please contact
W. W. Norton Special Sales at specialsales@wwnorton.com or 800-233-4830

Manufacturing by Sheridan
Book design by Lovedog Studio
Production manager: Julia Druskin

ISBN 978-0-87140-446-6

Liveright Publishing Corporation, 500 Fifth Avenue, New York, N.Y. 10110
www.wwnorton.com

W. W. Norton & Company Ltd., 15 Carlisle Street, London W1D 3BS

1 2 3 4 5 6 7 8 9 0

This book is dedicated in loving memory to our mothers,
Beatrice Gutmann and Zerka T. Moreno

CONTENTS

Introduction

A DUTY TO TELL

"Everybody Wants to Go to Heaven, but Nobody Wants to Die" is the title of an old blues song that captures the ironic way American society has come to view the afterlife, an ideal place where no one has to pay the price of achieving eternal perfection. In reality, though, our life choices test how much we are willing to pay. For health care, the stakes are high: longevity, the quality of life, and often life itself. When the stakes are so high only the best will do, but "the best" has to compete with all the expenses and other hard choices involved in getting the best.

To take the most glaring example, there's no limit on health care spending in the United States. We spend far more per capita on health care and medical science than any other society, an amount that continues to grow. If the results corresponded to the spending, there would be little reason to complain. Unfortunately, all that money hasn't made us the world's healthiest country—far from it. Compared to the populations of other high-income countries, Americans today have among the lowest life expectancy and the highest infant mortality. The United States spends about twice as much per capita on medical care as other affluent countries, providing insurance to a lower proportion of its population. American health care is inefficient and inequitable, the worst of both worlds.

Technological innovations coupled with other societal changes raise other hard questions—for example, about new means of human reproduction and their implications for the well-being of children,

as well as the liberty, responsibility, and sometimes even the iden-
tification of parents. The health and longevity for which we strive
have never come without public controversy, while also creating
tough choices among competing values. We must face up to the
fact that spending more on health care—both as a society and as
individuals—means spending less on something else we value, like
child care; elementary, secondary, or higher education; public or private transportation; housing; or discretionary quality-of-life goods
and services. Those hard choices are inevitable, and the costs aren't
only financial. Whether exemplified by divides over universal health
care insurance, investments in public health and mental health, new
reproductive technologies, genetic engineering, end-of-life care, or
organ donations, making health care choices for ourselves and our
society tests our priorities, our moral values, and our willingness to
work out our disagreements.

There are also rare and remarkable times when we actually serve
up the best and don't feel any need to do tough thinking about trade-
offs. As we were writing this book we were transfixed by the rescue
of a Thai youth soccer team and their young assistant coach from the
cave that flooded and trapped them for over two weeks. Hundreds
of rescuers from around the world were mobilized, from Thai Navy
Seals to an international group of volunteers. Once rescued, the team
and coach were helicoptered to the nearest city's hospital quaran-
tine for a week. No expense was spared; no knowledge or expertise
untapped. A volunteer diver heroically lost his life early in the rescue
operation.

What makes situations like these so exceptional? The life-and-death
stakes are immediate. The lives are identifiable and we positively
relate to them. We are conditioned to "think fast" rather than to
"think slow," as psychologist Daniel Kahneman puts it, springing
into action, sparing no expense, and doing everything we can to
come to the rescue. This happily turned out not to be a case of "lifeboat ethics," which asks who should live if not all can be saved. Yet
health care versions of lifeboat ethics occur daily in the United States

and worldwide for thousands who hope they will be selected for a scarce, lifesaving organ and who are not so prominently identifiable.

Human psychology is geared to identifiable victims in need of rescue. Most of what produces the everyday health care we need, however, is the product of thinking slow and making the hard choices that bring about longer, healthier lives for everyone. Contrast the Thai rescue, where nobody questioned whether it was worth the all-in cost of rescuing thirteen people, to the U.S. Congress's unwillingness to fund health insurance for all Americans, and to what happens every day in the United States with respect to health care for millions of low-income, vulnerable residents of our country. How much health care spending in the United States is consumed by emergency room visits is a matter of debate (somewhere between 2 and 10 percent), but even if we knew the exact amount, would anyone want to deny true emergency care, even at the risk of some people using the ER for routine care? Going all out in emergency situations is a testament to human compassion, but routinely using the emergency room to care for millions of uninsured is evidence of a wasteful, inhumane health care system. We want to explore how in normal times, when the stakes are extremely high for millions of people but not so immediately obvious, we can ethically address health care's hard choices.

In ages past, when it came to longevity and health, people usually had little choice and so turned their eyes skyward, hoping for the best. Today, by contrast, medical science's power for good is vastly greater than even just a century ago. Infectious diseases like polio, smallpox, measles, mumps, and diphtheria then were common killers. Now vaccinations and antibiotics have either eradicated or radically decreased their incidence. Even more significant are public health measures like clean water, regular food supplies, and other environmental improvements that with antibiotics and science-based therapies for diseases like stroke, cancer, and heart disease have created remedies that would have seemed like science fiction only a century ago. To take just one familiar measure of life expectancy change over the past century: an American born in the early twenty-first century is likely to live to eighty, whereas one born in 1900 had a life expectancy of only forty-seven years.

All stages of our lives are caught up in challenging ethical questions raised by modern medicine, health care, public health, and life science research. Here's just a sampling of the bioethical issues that we raise: Do we want to live in a society that nudges us toward greater public health by incentivizing the healthier among our choices? And if so, how do we want to be nudged and by whom? What legal means would we support to enable individuals to exercise more control over their deaths as well as their lives? As we are all able to live both longer and healthier lives, who should receive and pay for what kind of health care? What responsibility should individuals and communities take for the health of one another and for future generations? When some lifesaving treatments like organ transplants are scarce, how should our society decide who gets access? Absent evidence of the efficacy of a treatment, when should experimentation on humans be permitted? Once a treatment is found to be effective, who should benefit and at what cost? Are any unacceptable lines crossed when human cells are placed in animal brains for basic medical research that could lead to treatments for serious diseases?

Answers to these kinds of questions can be lifesaving, life extending, and life enhancing, or they may hasten the end of life or diminish its quality. That's why we think it's so important to attend to the ethics of health care, public health, and life sciences research—the field known as bioethics. Bioethics involves high stakes for everyone and requires informed reasoning, not heartless rationality. Not merely an individual enterprise but a social one, it also calls on us to think through issues together. When we work to improve medical care and advance medical science, we create a more moral politics that relies upon our collectively search for a common good.

Bioethics emerged in the decades after World War II just as medicine and medical science were experiencing rapid progress, creating new opportunities and challenges for the health care system. Bioethicists have articulated and applied principles to address the moral problems that emerged from this new landscape. Often they are also actively involved in moving that conversation forward. Not just the calling of a multidisciplinary group of professional experts, bioethics is also a social project that by its very nature engages us all. Exploring what's at stake in how the United States has handled a wide range of bioethical issues, we hope to encourage everyone to address these issues for yourselves, your families, communities, and society.

Although our focus is mainly on bioethics and the transformation of health care in America, bioethics has become a global field of interest. The problems of greatest concern vary depending on the region. In poorer countries, the demands of public health—such as clean water, nutrition, and vaccination programs—typically attract more attention than some of the high-technology concerns, such as in vitro fertilization and gene editing. Yet the bioethical principles we discuss shape the public dialogue even in the most impoverished areas where, for example, individual freedom or autonomy is invoked in support of the equal rights of women to control their sexual lives. And as the recent decrease in life expectancy in the United States suggests, millions of Americans may stand to benefit from our society paying greater attention to public health. The convergence across boundaries of why people care about bioethics has become at least as impressive as the differences.

The stories we tell in the next few pages help to explain why we care so much about bioethics. Everyone has vitally important stories like the ones that drew us together to write this book. Over the course of the last half century, as bioethics has grown in prominence, more people have come to believe in and practice patient-centered medicine. We begin by sharing two of our earliest personal memories about medical crises in our families. Our stories exemplify the fact that important experiences of patients and families have not always been appreciated. While we wrote this book entirely together, we include our two separate voices in this introduction in telling our personal stories that illustrate the many issues that contributed to our collaboration on this book.

AMY REMEMBERS

The first thing I noticed was the smell. The next thing I learned was that it was gangrene.

From the mid- to late 1950s, my mother, the late Beatrice Gutmann, and I would regularly drive from what my New York City cousins called the "country"—a small town in New York's Hudson River Valley called Monroe—to Long Island City in Queens, just across the East River, to visit my grandmother. An immigrant who spoke Yiddish and English, with a decidedly Yiddish accent, Eva Brenner was a strong, warm, and gregariously independent woman. As a ten-year-old only child, I relished running errands with her because she would strike up conversations and introduce me to more people over the course of a few city blocks than I could meet within miles of my country home.

Certain smells always linger from childhood and in my grandmother's tiny apartment it was the irresistible aroma of her homemade cookies. But not this time, when the smell led immediately to my grandmother lying in obvious distress on her opened Castro Convertible sofa bed, her right lower leg appearing profoundly swollen. I knew she took insulin for her type 2 diabetes, but she always seemed so upbeat that I hadn't thought that there was any cause for serious concern. My parents' greatest concern, I had thought, was being able to pay her bills so she'd feel secure. Now, all of a sudden, we were fearful for her life and afraid of losing her. My mother called for an ambulance.

At the hospital, the doctor told my mother that amputating her mother's leg was her only hope of surviving. He asked for my mother's permission. Taken aback by his request, she told the doctor that he needed Eva's permission to amputate her leg. Although Eva was in pain, she was fully conscious and capable of understanding the situation. She needed to decide whether to have her leg amputated in order to save her life. At my mother's insistence, the doctor reluctantly explained the dire situation to my grandmother, who consented and survived the operation. Nonetheless, Eva died just a few days later.

My mother later told me that, whatever the outcome, she would never have forgiven herself had she not insisted that the doctor let Eva decide for herself whether to undergo the leg amputation. As it turned out, this was to be the last decision of Eva's life. As obvious as a leg amputation under these circumstances might have seemed to many others, my mother knew that she couldn't simply assume that Eva would want to live without a leg.

Losing my only living, and immensely loving, grandparent was a life-transforming experience. It imprinted the painful reality of death and the preciousness of life on my consciousness from very early in my life. Even more distinctly, my mother's character was revealed with utmost clarity, because I realized then how she treated everyone with the respect they deserved—which meant, when necessary, not being unduly deferential to authority.

Much later in life, I learned that what had shocked my mother about her encounter with the emergency room doctor was, in fact, commonplace in medicine at the time. If you were a doctor in the late 1950s, you might well have turned to a textbook called *Medical Ethics*, published in 1956. Case 10 is entitled "Concealing the Nature of His [sic] Disease from a Patient."

> Miss A has chondrosarcoma [a form of cancer]. "Tell me," she pleads with Dr. B, "do I really have a cancer?" Dr. B, knowing that Miss A has ample time in which to prepare for death and wishing to spare her needless mental suffering, answers, "Your pains are due to arthritis."

Here's the textbook's ethics advice to Dr. B. It's probably not what you would expect:

> If Miss A actually has arthritis, or if Dr. B is convinced that everyone at her age does have at least a mild case of arthritis, his answer is not morally wrong.

The book then provides an "explanation" for this surprising conclusion:

> Dr. B does not affirm that Miss A's pains are due *solely* to arthritis. If she does have arthritis even in a mild form, Dr. B is justified in thinking that her pain is due in part to the arthritis, and hence his answer is not a lie. If Miss A really wanted the entire truth, she would ask, "Are *all* my pains due to arthritis?" In such cases patients often do not wish to pursue the matter preferring to accept an answer which leaves them with some ray of hope, even though in their hearts they know what the facts are. (Italics in the original.)

JONATHAN REMEMBERS

When I discovered the case of Miss A in the old textbook, I did a double take. In 1957, just a year after that medical ethics book was published, my forty-year-old mother, Zerka Moreno, was diagnosed with a chondrosarcoma, a rare kind of cancer that attacks the bone and the soft tissue that surrounds it. I was five. By the time of her diagnosis she had been suffering for a year with a growing, egg-shaped lump in her right shoulder. My parents concealed their anxiety from me. My one most vivid memory is sitting in the waiting area of a spa while my mother was getting a massage for what a physician told her was arthritis, a theory that the masseuse found implausible.

I have used the case of Miss A in my bioethics course at Penn for many years. Was Dr. B obligated to tell his patient that she had a cancer? After a bit of hedging, my students' responses are practically unanimous: of course, he should tell her the truth. For most of them it doesn't seem like a hard call. But when the author goes on to give the answer to the dilemma that the case implicitly creates for Dr. B, it is not what my students expect. They look at the question of truth telling in medical care through a twenty-first-century lens, not one grounded in the 1950s. But a mid-twentieth-century physician would have found the underlying rationale for withholding the truth familiar. The "therapeutic privilege" or "therapeutic exception" held that it is often ethically permitted and even necessary to withhold bad news so as not to upset the patient when, after all, there was nothing to be done anyway. In effect, the therapeutic privilege gave medical doctors a license to conceal, deceive, and lie, suspending an ancient moral premise about "bearing false witness." No other profession—such as accountants or lawyers, for example—had that privilege nor certainly did people have it in their personal lives. These were not "white lies" about trivial matters, but more often intentional silences, deceptions revolving around considerations of life-and-death decisions.

We have independent reason to believe that the textbook's analysis of the case of Miss A was not an outlier. In 1961 *JAMA* (*Journal of the American Medical Association*) published a survey that found that the vast majority of doctors who responded rarely or never disclosed a cancer diagnosis. Among their conclusions: "Euphemisms are the general rule"; "The modal policy is to tell as little as possible in the most general terms consistent with maintaining cooperation in treatment"; and "The vast majority of these doctors feel that almost all patients really do not want to know regardless of what people say." Yet the number of doctors who said they would want to be told if they had such a diagnosis was far greater than the number who said they would tell their patients.

In my mother's case the truth was not concealed and ultimately couldn't be. The tumor in her shoulder was indeed life-threatening. After a fruitless round of radiation therapy at Memorial Hospital in New York City, she agreed to an amputation of her right arm at the clavicle. However, her story had another couple of twists. My father was a famous psychiatrist. While my mother was in the hospital receiving radiation therapy, my dad walked into her room. They were alone. He wandered over to the window, looked into the middle distance, and made some small talk. As he never made small talk, my mother knew something was up. Finally, he told her that an amputation was necessary. At this revelation, she was actually relieved. The fact that a "brother physician" was assumed to be the suitable person to disclose this information says much about the era.

A few months later, my mother was looking for something in my father's night table. Crumpled up at the back of the drawer was a letter to him on her surgeon's letterhead. The note reminded him that if her cancer didn't recur within five years, they could consider her cured. This was news to her as that was not a conversation the surgeon had ever had with my mother. Here was the therapeutic privilege at work in yet another form. Of course, I was too young to understand any of this at the time. Young children, both then and now, have a hard time conceptualizing death, but they can understand the loss of a body part. My dad carefully explained to me that my mother would come home from the hospital without an arm. Being a young child, I asked whether I would see blood.

A DUTY TO TELL

It's rare for anyone to reach adulthood without experiencing a death or serious illness in their family. Yet for nearly all of human history, people died at home. Millions of people now die in institutions, such as nursing homes and hospitals. This major change alone has meant both that many of us are less familiar with the dying process itself and that when death does come, it's often preceded by treatments that involve some combination of advanced technology, complex surgery, and sophisticated drugs. These same factors also have created ethical problems that would have astonished our great grandparents.

Eva and Zerka faced their medical crises just a few years before generational changes transformed the contours of the ethics underlying modern medicine. For generations, doctors concealed rather than told the truth as best they knew it from their patients. As outlined in the Hippocratic oath and other classic statements of ethics for physicians, a doctor's duties included confidentiality and concern for their patients' well-being. But a duty to tell patients the truth about their ailments was *not* among them. What prevailed was "the silent world of doctor and patient," according to psychiatrist and legal scholar Jay Katz, in which the hidden was often more important than what was disclosed. "At least since Hippocratic days," Katz writes, "patients have been asked to trust their physicians without question. But only in recent years have doctors been asked to trust patients by conversing with them about medical options and soliciting their views on how to proceed." For reasons we will explore, the one-way discourse between doctors and patients that Katz describes began to be replaced by a preponderance of more diverse and disparate voices in the 1960s and 1970s. This was a turning point in medical ethics that separated the old "doctor ethics" from the new bioethics that championed a duty to tell the truth (which we call the "duty to tell" for short).

The duty to tell was often not implemented well and certainly wasn't accepted or implemented everywhere. Great shortcomings remain in the now-mandated practice known as "informed consent," but it is far more developed and widely practiced than it was in our childhoods. The duty to tell is also not accepted in all parts of the world or in all cultures. Many still insist, for example, that it is better for people not to know bad news. But the duty to tell the truth is, generally speaking, an internationally acknowledged standard for doctor-patient and researcher-research participant relations. Individuals shouldn't be forced to know what they don't wish to learn, but it's very clear that the ethics widely governing health care today requires that the truth—not lies or deceptive omissions—be told as long as that truth is relevant to a patient's health care and her decision making. Any exceptions require strong overriding reasons. In the cases of Eva and Zerka, no overriding reasons justified withholding the truth, curtailing their ability to chart their lives in light of the truth.

A duty to tell was just the beginning. A responsibility to listen to what patients have to say remains an essential work in progress. Yet listening not only shows respect for patients, it is critically important for accurate diagnoses and effective treatments, something that punishing clinical schedules miserably fail to appreciate. In this respect, the pressures of modern medical practice appear to have caused the art of listening to lose ground. Taking a thorough history, after all, remains a core requirement of the skilled clinician. Much to the frustration of many clinicians, actually listening to patients challenges the financial imperatives that demand that doctors now see as many patients as possible. And "seeing" patients also competes with the ubiquitous screens in the modern consulting room. Taking the considerable time needed to enter and read data on those screens, doctors might miss important nonverbal cues that can be key to a diagnosis. In the coming years, more of those screens will also display information from complex algorithms, which analyze vast quantities of data drawn from millions of people and apply those data to individual patients. Ironically, patients may feel this "personalized" medicine to be rather impersonal. Learning how best to treat patients by listening to and seeing them as well as applying internet-derived data vividly illustrate how solving important bioethical problems involves integrating so many disciplines, including the psychology of communication, the economics and politics of health care systems, and even cyber-culture.

Modern bioethics has matured into a field that extends well beyond the ethics of clinical medicine into public health, human experiments, genetics, neuroscience, and many other fields. And accordingly, our book is not a comprehensive account of bioethics but one that charts its evolution over our lifetimes and gives the reader our shared sense of its remarkable breadth and complexity. We believe every reader has their own favorite story, historical analogy, or fascinating issue that we will not have mentioned. Our goal is to stimulate conversation and discovery about some important matters of our health care and our humanity that we all face. Otherwise those matters will be decided for us without our informed individual or collective consent.

HARD CHOICES

We have encountered these issues in our public as well as in our personal lives. We spent seven years together on President Obama's

Presidential Commission for the Study of Bioethical Issues (Amy as chair, Jonathan as senior advisor), publicly deliberating over dozens of other controversial issues of health care, public health, and cutting-edge research that deeply engaged a broad public. Before that, we had spent thirty years as participants in bioethics debates, Amy as a political philosopher and Jonathan as a historian. We thought that together we could write a far richer account of the rise of bioethics and the transformation of American health care than we could separately.

Bioethical issues today are about all stages of life, from conception through death. They even reach into the future of humanity, due to remarkable advances in fields like genetics, where reengineering the basic building blocks of life is no longer a distant fantasy. Most of these issues confront us not only as individuals and families but also as interconnected citizens of our society and the world. Agonizing individual decisions, such as whether to extend or terminate a loved one's life support, often make the headlines. We have too often neglected the societal dimensions of our bioethical choices. Those dimensions, which have become a focus of *Everybody Wants to Go to Heaven, but Nobody Wants to Die*, include engaging diverse communities in constructive conversations, understanding our competing perspectives, and justifying public decisions to better achieve some common good, often amid controversy.

Our hard choices and our public controversies typically reflect competing values and goals. A persistent challenge in the pursuit of promising medical research, for example, is not to let the goal of maximizing social welfare override respect for human rights. Research participants must not be subject to disproportionate risks, and their informed consent must be obtained. We faced this challenge in high relief on the bioethics commission when we were asked to recommend whether the U.S. government should start testing an anthrax vaccine on children. The vaccine, which had been found safe for adults, had not yet been found safe to use on children. Imposing unknown risks on a relatively small number of children as research subjects, who are themselves unlikely to benefit from the vaccine, promised large social gains in protecting millions of children in the future. Parents, pediatricians, national security experts, and others offered conflicting advice on how best to proceed. By openly addressing the competing claims, the commission's deliberations were instrumental to our arriving at and publicly defending the recommendations that we discuss in chapter 6.

We set out to engage readers in a wide range of bioethical issues that confront American society. Part I chronicles a remarkable cultural transformation over the past sixty years from "doctor knows best" to a patient-centered view of American health care. Many more patients' voices entered into health care debates, as bioethics emerged and expanded its public engagement. Too often neglected, and one focus of our attention, is America's underinvestment in public health and mental health. Part II confronts some major controversies with life-and-death stakes, sometimes for only a few people but often for millions. These include ongoing debates over physician-assisted death, affordable universal health insurance, and organ transplants. Part III and the epilogue turn to the choices posed by new medical technologies, such as gene editing, synthetic biology, and brain imaging, that create exciting opportunities and mind-boggling challenges, some so profound that they call into question the very nature of our human identity. Taken together, these issues leave much room for debate, but no room to doubt the impact of bioethical decisions on the quality of all of our lives. That is why we care, and why, we believe, others should care passionately as well.

Part One

NEW
VOICES

One

CHANGING
TIMES

O ver the second half of the twentieth century, Americans witnessed a historic change from an ethics that accepted paternalistic, doctor-oriented medicine into one prescribing a doctor-patient
dialogue. Gone are the centuries when doctors often avoided disclosing a poor prognosis, as when Amy's mother was asked to sign
the consent form for Amy's grandmother or when Jonathan's mother
wasn't told the details about her prospects for a cure. The medical
profession no longer endorses these deceptions or omissions, and the
patient public no longer tolerates them. It's remarkable how quickly
the old medical ethics shifted to the new bioethics of truth telling.
An observer transported suddenly from the 1950s might think that
modern bioethics bootstrapped itself into being after centuries of
"doctor knows best." But many variables converged, leading to the
collapse of medical paternalism and to the rise of a bioethics capable
of addressing rapidly changing times.

That physicians had long been given some degree of implicit permission to mislead, if not to lie outright, tells us something about
historic expectations for doctor-patient relationships. Disclosing less
than the whole truth about a patient's condition made some sense in
the nineteenth and early twentieth centuries, when the shift from the
old medical arts to the new science-based medicine was still unfolding. Even the much-admired Hippocratic oath says nothing about
telling patients the truth. Yet the common practice not merely of non-

disclosure but of lying and deception persisted even into the twentieth century as the science of medicine had far more to offer. Why?

The continued acceptance of this ethics exception had much to do with the prestige of the medical profession. Between World War II and the 1960s, American medicine in many ways came into a golden age. The Vietnam War and the Watergate scandal had not yet undermined Americans' faith or at least our trust in institutions. Admiration of the medical profession and of medical science was at an all-time high. Penicillin was discovered in 1928, vanquishing diseases that had plagued human beings since before recorded history. The first antibiotic had justly been hailed as a "magic bullet," but it took another twenty years for penicillin to become widely available. After running well-publicized trials in the early 1950s, the polio vaccine was widely distributed, a cure for yet another disease that devastated generations. CPR—cardiopulmonary resuscitation—saved lives. Thanks in large measure to improved diets and sanitation, most Americans lived longer. The government invested in medical research as never before. People had more reason to trust the continued progress of medicine and public health and the expertise of doctors.

NOT SO HAPPY DAYS

From small towns to big cities, doctors in the 1950s acquired an elevated social standing. Where once they could at best predict the course of an illness and suggest ways to manage symptoms, now they could actually prescribe a cure. Growing up in the 1950s just a few miles from each other in New York's Hudson River valley, we both have fond memories of our doctors. We saw them as wise counselors who provided comfort, dispensed wisdom, and even gave suggestions about colleges and career paths as they made house calls armed with little more than their obligatory black bag, setting off afterward to the next patient, often in the pitch of night.

Health care, however, wasn't very expensive. In 1950, health care hovered around 4.5 percent of the U.S. gross domestic product. It is now about 18 percent and growing. In the first decades after World War II, it seemed that we could get to heaven without paying for it, or at least without paying much. Most working people received health insurance through employment-based programs. The unemployed relied on family or charity or the forgiveness of hospital and doctor bills. Many thought that the next step after social security in 1935 would be some kind of government-provided health insurance, in the spirit of President Franklin Roosevelt's liberal New Deal. Starting in 1960, some of the indigent elderly did receive a modest amount of government health care coverage, but not many. The medical historian Rosemary Stevens has written that "in the early 1960s, the choices for uninsured or underinsured elderly patients needing hospital service were to spend their savings, rely on funding from their children, seek welfare (and the social stigma this carried), hope for charity from the hospitals, or avoid care altogether."

The passage of Medicare in 1965 greatly reduced these stresses on older Americans, but Medicaid created an entirely different narrative. Tens of millions of low-income Americans who might have qualified for Medicaid remained uninsured. Rules for access to Medicaid still vary widely from one state to another. Even in the case of Medicare, the medical profession did its best to prevent its passage. In order to pass Medicare and also to preempt a potential boycott by the highly organized medical profession, especially the powerful American Medical Association (AMA), Congress finally passed legislation that maintained fee-for-service payments in its reimbursement structure for American health care goods and services. These new laws incentivized expensive hospital and surgical procedures and helped to underwrite costly advances in medical technology, making the United States a leader in those achievements but not in affordable or universal access to basic medical care.

While Medicare and Medicaid increased affordable access to millions of previously uninsured Americans, millions of children, parents, and other working women and men were still left uninsured for even basic care. Largely by dint of the incentives built into its fee-for-service and reimbursement structure, Medicare and Medicaid were partly responsible for major cost escalations in health care for everyone, for incentivizing specialization in medical education, and ironically for undermining the once widespread assumption that health care was destined to become more and more affordable and accessible in America. With rising costs came declining public satisfaction, and as Paul Starr writes in his classic *The Social Transformation of American Medicine*, "Medicine, like many other American institutions, suffered a stunning loss of confidence in the 1970s."

Over the ensuing decades, as the medical economist Rashi Fein has shown, medical costs escalated at historically high rates. Writing in 1988, Fein warned that without national health insurance, "We can expect additional pressure to restrict existing health insurance policies, to increase patient 'cost-sharing,' and to cut benefits. More and more of us will be forced into health plans and patterns of care we now reject. It will become harder to pay for the care we need." At the same time, access to primary care doctors, nurses, and trust in the medical profession (as well as in most other professions) precipitously declined. Only 34 percent of Americans in 2012 said they had great confidence in the leaders of the medical profession, as compared to 73 percent in 1966.

CHANGING TIMES

Another sea change took place in doctor-patient relations, one measurable in the same terms as that 1961 *JAMA* survey that showed that the vast majority of doctors were comfortable exercising their therapeutic privilege and concealing cancer diagnoses from their patients. In 1979, *JAMA* published a new survey that asked the same question. This time, nearly all the doctors said they did use the word "cancer" with their patients. This remarkable cultural shift took less than two decades. Few drastic changes in long-standing attitudes happen so quickly, especially in a profession that has been around for about as long as human beings have gotten sick. What happened?

The answer is complicated but includes some events that shook Americans' confidence in the seemingly limitless possibilities of medical science and the prerogatives of its practitioners. First, although the 1965 Medicare and Medicaid laws expanded access to both low-income and older Americans, major gaps in coverage for tens of millions remained, health care costs were escalating, and the lack of affordable high-quality health care—especially to those who remained uninsured—was obvious. Second, Americans began to see that the ethics of health care is not and must not be primarily a doctor's ethics but rather it must be an ethics of, by, and for patients, their families, and the broader citizenry. These two growing sensibilities moved many issues surrounding sickrooms into classrooms and helped give rise to modern-day bioethics.

The black bag-toting, house-calling family doctor, a source of authority in whom many Americans had once placed considerable trust, was starting to feel nostalgic. Changing attitudes emerged in popular culture, especially in the television shows about physicians. *Marcus Welby, M.D.* ran from 1969 to 1976, its popularity based partly on the man who played its lead character, the comforting 1950s *Father Knows Best* actor Robert Young. Portrayed as a compassionate and wise doctor who regularly made house calls, Dr. Welby employed unorthodox treatments to solve tangled medical and human problems. He figured out potentially devastating situations involving depression, brain damage, learning disabilities, leprosy, emphysema, mononucleosis, rabies, a flu epidemic, a fatal form of sclerosis, and ulcers—all in his second season alone (when the show topped the Nielsen ratings in prime time). In subsequent seasons, Dr. Welby's "solutions" included urging a depressed middle-aged man to resist his homosexual impulses, provoking hurls of protest from gay activists. An episode aired that conflated homosexuality with pedophilia, leading sponsors, even then, to pull advertising and seventeen network affiliates to refuse airing the episode. By the end of its largely successful run, *Marcus Welby* seemed a throwback to a less complicated time, although in fact it was a time that never really existed.

As early as the first season of *Marcus Welby*, economists were noting the uptick in health care costs. In an experiment to see whether this increasing medical inflation could be brought under control, President Nixon signed a bill in 1973 promoting health care maintenance organizations (HMOs). To deliver quality health care at a lower price, HMO doctors had to be more aware of the costs of care as well as more sensitive to the demands of patients increasingly referred to as consumers of health care. Dr. Welby had no such constraints. Like the kindly doctors of our childhoods, Dr. Welby felt free to dispense advice without having to account for his unreimbursed time or worry about his malpractice insurance. But by the series' end, he seemed to be basking more in the nostalgic glow of the 1950s rather than reflecting the less telegenic but increasingly dominant complexities of the late 1970s medical world.

Comparing portrayals of physicians and the hospital environment in the early 1960s to the early 1970s reveals contrasts. Not long after President Kennedy was inaugurated, two charismatic young TV doctors vied for America's attention: the sprightly, handsome Dr. James Kildare and the darkly brooding Dr. Ben Casey. Although they encountered all sorts of obstacles in their urban hospitals, they both pursued the care of their patients with unquestioned commitment and idealistic verve. In that spirit, each was supported by a wise, elderly white male mentor who represented the medical establishment: Dr. Gillespie for Kildare and Dr. Zorba for Casey.

One notable exception to the white male-dominated world of TV medicine was *Julia*, which ran for three seasons starting in 1968. Diahann Carroll led the cast as a super competent, multitasking, beautiful African American nurse, a single mother who had lost her husband in Vietnam. Her mentor, the craggy Dr. Chegley, had no patience for racism but a proud preference for "pretty" nurses. Julia's single-parenting challenges get more airtime than her expert nursing, as undervalued by the media as by the health care system. And despite the show's intended message of racial equality, Julia is scripted to play out her struggles as a nurse and mother with the requisite sit-com lightheartedness of the day.

Other women in medical dramas in the 1960s were given support-ing roles. Even the attempted exceptions—a female doctor originally played alongside Ben Casey—ended up proving the rule that women had less power, prestige, and pay than white men, and powerful men of color were largely unseen. Dr. Maggie Graham was to become Dr. Casey's romantic interest, but the writers failed to figure out how to make that work. She was transferred from anesthesiology into neu-rology so she would appear on screen less often. The show was also exceptional in employing a registered nurse, Alice Rodriguez, as its primary technical advisor, yet she received no screen credit for this role. The "primal metaphysics" opening of the show, which featured Dr. Zorba's hand drawing the symbols on a chalkboard for Man, Woman, Birth, Death, and Infinity, was as "deep" as a 1960s network television series dared to pretend to be. Culturally defiant it was not.

Yet in 1971 a film called *The Hospital* featured an exhausted, sui-cidal, and sexually impotent successor to Gillespie and Zorba. Play-ing hospital director Dr. Herbert Bock, George C. Scott delivered what is generally considered one of the great monologues in movie history, decrying "the most enormous medical entity ever con-ceived"—which transplants organs, manufactures genes, and con-ceives of cloning people—yet presides over a society where "people are sicker than ever!" Dr. Bock's sexual inadequacy is a metaphor for a once promising scientist who is desperately struggling to save his embattled and resource-starved city hospital from a suspicious minority community, money-grubbing surgeons, and a city govern-ment that would prefer to ignore the place. From his office window, in a drunken fury, he delivers a tirade against the medical establish-ment and society's failure to protect its most vulnerable. It is a cry of pain and defeat—a long way from the world of *Marcus Welby*.

So was the perpetually underfinanced, run-down hospital in the 1980s show *St. Elsewhere*, staffed by some brilliant and dedicated doctors and some who failed to make the grade either morally or medically. Ten years later, *ER*'s central character, Dr. Doug Ross, played by George Clooney, also has a complex personal life but remains determined to give his patients the best care possible regardless of the rules. In the first decade of the twenty-first century, Dr. Gregory House became even more rebellious. Continuing the post-1960s theme of the personally flawed physician, he was addicted to pain medication.

As was Jackie Peyton, brilliantly portrayed by Edie Falco in the lead role of *Nurse Jackie* from 2009 to 2015. Jackie works as an emergency room nurse with enormous compassion and expertise, but highly questionable ethics (driven to the ground by her addiction), in the underfunded, overburdened, and bureaucratized environment of a New York City hospital. Her addiction begins with chronic back pain, which afflicts nurses more than any other profession. Both Jackie's personal and professional life poignantly degenerate over a series ironically entered for awards' purposes as a comedy. Falco won the Emmy as best comedy actress in 2010 for what media critic Eric Deggans aptly praised as "tv's most honest depiction of addiction."

If *House* and *Nurse Jackie* anticipated public distress about an opioid epidemic, Dr. Shaun Murphy in *The Good Doctor* more recently captured the fascination with spectrum disorders (in his case autism), while demonstrating the medical insight of a savant. Each reflected the spirit of the time without the comfort zones available in the imagination of post–World War II America.

THE "BIOETHICIST"

As America entered the later 1960s and early 1970s, traditional institutions, both religious and secular, declined as sources of moral authority. Amid all the uncertainty, a new role—the "bioethicist"— emerged. Bioethicists did not try to fill the void of declining religious or secular medical authorities, but they did speak directly to a growing concern about the ethics of medicine and the politics of health care. In fact, the study of medical ethics is about as old as medicine, just as the Hippocratic oath suggests. But bioethics today is different from the traditional study of medical ethics. Traditional medical ethics was ethics for doctors, like Healy's 1956 textbook. There was little or no decision-making role for patients, as both our family experiences attest.

When Katz described the traditional one-sided doctor-patient encounter, his psychoanalytic orientation emphasized the inadequacies of the relationship, each side projecting its assumptions and expectations on the other. Nonetheless, he was able to cite the history of legal cases that suggested how society's expectations about that relationship had been changing since the late nineteenth century as medicine was becoming more of a science and less of an art. Both British and American courts were gradually hearing complaints from patients who believed that they were inappropriately treated. Many of these cases involved surgery, perhaps because in those instances the damage done to the patient was particularly obvious.

Among the most famous of these cases was one that took place at New York Hospital in 1908, when a patient consented to an examination for a fibroid tumor but had previously refused to have the tumor removed. The surgeon removed the tumor anyway while the patient was under anesthesia. In 1914 the New York State Court of Appeals ruled against the hospital with this ringing statement:

> Every human being of adult years and sound mind has a right to determine what shall be done with his own body; and a surgeon who performs an operation without his patient's consent commits an assault, for which he is liable in damages.

It was a historic endorsement of patient rights, but, as Katz noted, it was toothless, as the court also found that because the hospital was a charitable institution, it wasn't responsible for its employees' (in this case the surgeon's) actions. This case was among a number that vindicated patients' rights in principle but without any real sanctions, leading Katz to conclude that the reality of the doctor-patient relationship was allowed to remain a largely silent one.

By the 1960s, however, at least two major social changes in medicine—its increasing cost and its growing power to produce predictable improvements in human health—changed the doctor-patient relationship itself. The struggle to determine how to modernize that relationship fueled the creation of the field of bioethics. A key element was the role of simply telling patients the truth, of opening up the silent space that Katz described. In the courts 1972 was a pivotal year, as three legal cases clearly established the duty of doctors to obtain informed consent from their patients. Coming one after the other in several jurisdictions, these cases represented a remarkable legal consensus that crystallized the changed attitudes about doctor-patient relations since the 1950s.

A related reason for bioethics bursting onto the scene was the public fascination with some major events reported in newly aggressive media beginning to question, ever so cautiously, some prevailing assumptions of the day, including the truthfulness and trustworthiness of many major institutions. Newspapers and magazines ramped up their engagement in investigative journalism and questioned previously sacrosanct assumptions not only about political institutions but also about infrequently questioned professions, including medicine. Newspapers published stories about unconsented experiments with debilitated, elderly patients and hepatitis experiments with profoundly disabled children, as well as the Tuskegee syphilis experiment in which hundreds of low-income African American men were observed, not informed of their disease, and not treated for decades. Katz closely examined these cases for their ethical failures. The new bioethicists found themselves in demand by the press to comment on the rapidly changing environment of medicine and ethics. And all of this was mainly taking place in the United States, a nation in an economically privileged and politically dominant position in the post–World War II era.

In response, the education of young doctors began to change. Historically, medical students learned their ethics by independent study or by their mentors' example. Sometimes a senior physician might give a lecture or two, often based on the Hippocratic oath. While the graduating class might recite the oath as a ritual before receiving their degrees, few medical leaders believed medical ethics to be an appropriate focus of either serious teaching or deep scholarship. Sensing that more needed to be said about medical ethics than they were taught in their classes, at graduation ceremonies in the later 1960s some medical classes modified the oath or substituted the prayer of Maimonides, written by a twelfth-century Jewish physician and philosopher. Many young doctors found their medical ethics education inadequate.

SEEKING "RELEVANCE"

While the medical students were focused on the demands of their grueling education, many of their campuses were sites of major demonstrations and even violence in protest of the Vietnam War. In the late 1960s and early 1970s, several medical schools, aware of the social turbulence, hired professors of medical ethics and established programs on ethics. Like their students, a new generation of medical school faculty believed that they needed to respond to the unfolding controversies about war and political scandal, and that response needed to be based on both publicly defensible facts and values. They, too, desired to be "relevant." Young leaders in academic medicine were energized by the new socially conscious atmosphere. Among them was Edmund Pellegrino, who held a vast range of important positions in his long career as an eminent physician-ethicist and may have done more to advance the cause of ethics in U.S. medical schools than any other individual. Under the influence of Pellegrino and others, some of the old land-grant universities, like the University of Texas in Galveston, had institutes on the history of medicine that gradually incorporated ethics. Theologians played a leading role in creating a new professional organization, the Society for Health and Human Values, which held annual meetings and published educational materials.

Other pioneers created whole organizations devoted to the study of bioethics. At Georgetown University, the Kennedy family, acting through its foundation, provided funds to establish the Kennedy Institute of Ethics. Despite their wealth and prominence, the Kennedys were no strangers to the battleground of medical ethics, when President Kennedy's older sister, Rosemary, who was born in 1918, became a victim of a psychosurgery gone wrong. One of nine children, Rosemary was intellectually disabled from birth, a problem that became more obvious as a teenager. Hoping to manage her moods and risk-taking behavior, her father, Joseph P. Kennedy, agreed to a fairly new procedure known as a prefrontal lobotomy, which involved severing some brain tissue. The results were catastrophic. Rosemary, who died at eighty-six, was unable to care for herself and was institutionalized for the rest of her life.

Devout Roman Catholics, the Kennedys were aware of the hard choices that pediatricians were making when they cared for sick babies. In 1971 the Kennedy Foundation sponsored an educational film called *Who Should Survive? One of the Choices on Our Conscience*. Inspired by actual cases at Johns Hopkins University, the film dealt with parents' decisions to let their infants born with Down syndrome—a genetic abnormality—die rather than have a straightforward surgery to correct an associated malformation that prevented them from eating. The cases frustrated and appalled Robert Cooke, the director of pediatrics at Johns Hopkins who knew that, with loving care and education, people with Down syndrome can lead satisfying lives. Yet he was unable to override the parents' decisions not to permit the surgery, thus dooming their babies to death. Angered that his hands were tied, he took his concerns to the Kennedy family, who sustained and financed his efforts. Their foundation supported the production of the film and the creation of the Kennedy Institute of Ethics.

At that same time, in 1969, philosopher Daniel Callahan and psychiatrist Willard Gaylin, neighbors in Hastings-on-Hudson, New York, decided to create a think tank independent of a university. Their plan grew out of a Christmas party conversation about advances in medicine and science that were challenging long-standing moral values. They had no money, only an exciting idea that seemed right for the times. Years later, they remembered calling up a few interesting people to attend some meetings in a rented space and in Callahan's home. Their efforts quickly caught the attention of a major foundation. Years later, whenever other ambitious people with few resources asked Callahan how they got started he simply said, "We just started!" Their struggle for a name reflected efforts to frame what they were up to. First it was a Center for the Study of Value and the Sciences of Man, then the Institute of Society, Ethics, and the Life Sciences. Fortunately, that mouthful morphed into simply the Hastings Center.

The Hastings Center and the Kennedy Institute were products of an era that challenged many traditional values. Like the doctors, the philosophers turned their intellectual attention to ethical issues raised by historic events and pressing contemporary problems. A new journal, *Philosophy & Public Affairs*, was "founded in the belief that a philosophical examination of . . . issues [of public concern] can contribute to their clarification and to their resolution." Its earliest contributors took strong and often opposing positions on issues, including abortion rights, the relevance of the Nuremberg trials, wartime justice, and famine amid affluence. Ethical inquiry in the academy broadened its scope, honoring its historical roots, dating back to Plato, by becoming more socially relevant in its contemporary ambitions. The intellectual environment in America was fertile for bioethics. A newly minted philosopher of science, Hastings scholar Arthur Caplan applied his background to the implications of sociobiology as well as issues like organ donation, the care of severely ill newborns, and human experiments. Women and minorities entered the field. Although almost all institutions were dominated by white males in those days, even more than today, bioethics in the 1970s did reflect the changing times. Patricia King, a pioneering black law professor at Georgetown University, served on the first national bioethics commission and later on a presidential commission that investigated human radiation experiments. Hastings Center scholar and philosopher Ruth Macklin led the way in addressing many emerging ethical issues, including research involving children and care for people with mental illness and intellectual disabilities, and later became president of the International Association of Bioethics.

Prominent scholars supplied philosophical fuel for public debate about the just distribution of health care. John Rawls's *A Theory of Justice*, published in 1971, was widely hailed as reviving the grand philosophical tradition. The philosopher and bioethicist Norman Daniels applied Rawls's principle of fair equality of opportunity in strong defense of equal access to the health care that people need to function normally. Meeting people's health care needs, Daniels argued, is a practical precondition for fair equality of opportunity and consistent with protecting everyone's equal basic liberties. The economist and philosopher Amartya Sen developed a distinctive "capability approach" and later became an influential champion of universal health care throughout the world, arguing that affordable health care is essential because it enables us to do all the other important things in our lives. These liberal philosophies all strongly support a universal human right to affordable health care.

In stark contrast and direct rebuttal to Rawls's *A Theory of Justice*, the libertarian philosopher Robert Nozick's (1974) *Anarchy, State and Utopia* defended the most minimal state that protects people only against violence, theft, and fraud. A night-watchman state does not distribute health care on the basis of need because taxing some people to aid others violates their natural right of freedom from interference. Distinctively and dramatically, such a single-valued libertarian perspective considers taxation for health care, even if democratically authorized, as tantamount to forced labor. It also "frees" doctors from any ethical obligation to help heal their patients. Doctors need to compete to obtain the consent of their patients through the marketplace. No value other than freedom of choice is considered obligatory or inherent in the ethical practice of medicine.

This debate between philosophers may strike many as too abstract and beside the point of what's really at stake for most people concerned about affordable health care. Yet it not only exposed what's ethically at stake in the practice of medicine, it also foreshadowed the highly polarized and consequential debate in contemporary American politics about affordable access to health care and health insurance. Rawls and Nozick, the liberal and the libertarian, respectively, revealed the theoretical roots of what has become a hyperpartisan divide between Democratic supporters and Republican opponents of a universal right to affordable health care. While universal health care is an "affordable dream" even for relatively poor countries like Thailand, Sri Lanka, Costa Rica, Cuba, and China, as Sen observes:

> The United States, which can certainly afford to provide health-care at quite a high level for all Americans, is exceptional in terms of the popularity of the view that any kind of public establishment of universal healthcare must somehow involve unacceptable intrusions into private life.

By the early 1980s, the American public experienced escalating health care costs and became acutely aware of the enormous life consequences of not being able to afford health care for themselves and their families. But affordable universal health care still did not become a universally shared dream among the American public.

In effect, the philosophical turn toward public affairs gave voice to the millions of people who could not afford access to health care through no fault of their own. This brought into sharp relief the difference between those who lacked basic opportunities in life because they could not afford health care and those with insurance-paying jobs or more money. In 1981, presenting his work to the President's Commission for the Study of Ethical Problems in Medicine and Biomedical and Behavioral Research, Daniels argued strongly for affordable access to health care as an essential condition for equal opportunity.

Whether affordable universal health care is considered essential to equal opportunity or as an essential enabler of all the other important things in life, it struggled in American politics to "be distinguished from the ethics of aiming at complete equality." For the goal of universal health care [UHC] to have a prayer in the United States, as Sen astutely notes, it must "be distinguished from the value of eliminating inequalities in general, which would demand much more radical economic and social changes than UHC requires." Universal health care does not restrict anyone's basic liberties since it still permits those with more money or additional insurance to obtain extra services.

In seeking to be socially relevant, bioethicists appreciate philosophical distinctions like this one that turn out to be practically important. The only hope of finding some common cause in defending universal health care in the United States across the political divides is to distinguish it from more comprehensive prescriptions to eliminate inequality. The libertarianism of the economist and philosopher F. A. Hayek, for example, favors providing "a comprehensive system of social insurance" for individuals while respecting their market freedom to buy more. Writing in the 1970s shortly after Rawls published his theory of justice, Hayek denounced the "mirage of social justice," a dangerous desire to impose comprehensive top-down redistribution schemes on society. But he consistently defended the compatibility between the state's providing social insurance to all and preserving individual freedom. As we see in chapter 5, this compatibility is roughly what's accepted by Americans who are willing to compromise across partisan lines.

PROFESSING BIOETHICS

In the changing times of the 1970s, the profession of bioethics emerged, and its practitioners challenged long-standing traditions, such as the therapeutic privilege of doctors and the failure of health systems to ensure affordable health care for all. But what gives anyone the right to profess bioethics as a vocation? Some critics derided the term "bioethicist" because they took the very word to suggest an ethical authority. Any term that suggests that any person has some special moral authority is bound to be suspect, all the more so at times when trust in almost all authority has dramatically declined.

Immersed in problems like what counts as informed consent to treatment, fairness in access to health care, or humane end-of-life care, bioethicists study and teach the subject matters of bioethics, just as philosophers study and teach philosophy and academic lawyers study and teach the law. For example, the strength of the ethical precept that everyone in the United States *ought* to have access to affordable health care depends on the possibility that everyone actually *can* be afforded such access and care. As the philosopher Immanuel Kant famously observed: *Ought implies can*. Just as understanding the "ought" of universal health care calls on moral and political philosophy, the "can" calls on knowledge of economics, political science, psychology, sociology, and the health care professions. Thus bioethics is a consummately multidisciplinary and collaborative field. Although it fits uneasily within any single discipline, bioethics resonates strongly with traditional philosophy's mission of addressing the controversial issues of its time.

Bioethics is not a secular priesthood. No professionals should be deemed morally virtuous at practicing what they teach simply by virtue of their intellectual and teaching expertise. Most self-identified bioethicists begin their research and teach moral or political philosophy, theology, or an academic profession like medicine, nursing, or engineering, but certainly not as substitutes for clergy or other moral mentors to whom people might look for guidance. Complicating the picture, many bioethicists are educated in religious traditions, but they, too, write for diverse audiences and not exclusively from a particular theological perspective.

Many lawyers, philosophers, theologians, doctors, nurses, humanists, social scientists, scientists, and more recently engineers and

neuroscientists have warmed to the role of bioethics teaching, researching, and advising. It is, as it should be, often impossible to tell when
those who practice bioethics are speaking from their home discipline
or from the broad multidisciplinary field called bioethics. This is one
of the reasons we find the work so exciting, that in a world so highly
specialized, a common language in the study of science and human
values emerged.

Probably no more than a few dozen people would have called themselves "bioethicists" in the late 1970s. Yet in retrospect, a need had
been identified for a new kind of public conversation about health
care, medical science, and technology, and the ethical challenges
and opportunities they presented for a society already struggling
with poverty amid affluence and a widespread sense of alienation
from authority. Bioethics emerged as a site for that conversation, a
conversation—sometimes contentious, often constructive, but never
boring—that has continued ever since.

Two

BIOETHICS
GOES PUBLIC

Which came first, the public's or the professors' fascination with bioethical issues? In fact, one fed off the other in the 1970s. As the public's interest in medicine increased, bioethics education moved from esoteric to mainstream. Courses in bioethics were sparse in the early 1970s, but by the early 1990s they became what bioethics pioneer Albert Jonsen called in *The Birth of Bioethics* "an established part of medical education." Since then, student interest and enrollments in bioethics education have skyrocketed. Many arts and sciences faculties have created bioethics majors and minors that enable all students, not only future health care professionals, to understand the enormous impact of biomedical decision making. And the public's imagination and concern have been fired by one controversy after another, usually with ancient roots but with a decidedly modern cast that presents novel complexities.

SCANDALS AND PRINCIPLES

In 1972 newspapers reported an experiment with hundreds of low-income African American men in Macon County, Alabama. Since the early 1930s, they had been part of a U.S. Public Health Service study of syphilis in the "Negro male." Among the outrages were that they had not been told that they had a sexually transmitted disease and that they were not provided penicillin when it became available after World War II. For years, a few members of Congress had been pressing for a national commission to establish ethical principles to govern human experiments. The syphilis study revelations were the tipping point. One congressional mandate to the National Commission for the Protection of Human Subjects of Biomedical and Behavioral Research in 1974 was that it "identify the basic ethical principles which should underlie the conduct of biomedical and behavioral research involving human subjects [and] develop guidelines which should be followed in such research." In its landmark *Belmont Report*, the commission called upon all individuals and institutions to adhere to three fundamental principles when conducting research using human subjects, each of which was flagrantly violated in the syphilis experiments: respect for persons, beneficence, and justice. These three principles remain the dominant framework for analyzing the ethics of any proposed human experiment and are referenced in federal regulations.

The outrageous story of those black men in Tuskegee shocked the public conscience and led to the *Belmont Report*. Both had immediate and lasting influence on the regulation of human experiments and on the field of bioethics. By publicly stating three high-level principles that must guide scientific research with human subjects, the commission made clear that good science must be ethically grounded. This seminal moment demonstrated why bioethics is valuable even if bioethical standards in themselves do not, and generally cannot, make anyone ethical. Bioethics clarifies and publicizes essential conditions for the ethical conduct of medicine and science.

Years before the *Belmont Report*, the philosopher responsible for the initial draft of the report, Tom Beauchamp, had already been working on a textbook with religious studies professor James Childress. In their *Principles of Biomedical Ethics* (1981), they elaborated four principles aimed at providing an ethical framework beyond human experiments: respect for autonomy, nonmaleficence, beneficence, and justice. Although sometimes humorously called the "bioethics mantra," these principles changed in their meaning over time, as Beauchamp and Childress expanded on their significance and constructively addressed critics. Few textbooks have had so great an influence on a field of study, and for so long.

Of the principles in the bioethics mantra, justice especially requires a health care system that is fair and affordable. As applied specifically to human experiments, justice means that volunteers must be fairly selected, so that people who are especially vulnerable to manipulation must not be used in studies simply because they are readily available. Justice also demands that research volunteers not be drawn from groups that are unlikely to benefit from the results, like the men in the syphilis study. For societies to justify devoting scarce public resources to biomedical research, they also must accept an obligation to provide fair access to the fruits of biomedical science. The decades-long transformation of health care in America has still not achieved that goal, and in some ways the United States is losing ground. In that sense, in the American context, justice is the least successful of the principles of bioethics, and the most urgent to attend to.

DAX'S CASE

People entering colleges and medical schools in the 1970s were familiar with the syphilis study and other highly publicized bioethics scandals. Some schools responded with new "experimental" courses on bioethics. At George Washington University, for example, the first hour of the course was given over to a film or lecture, the second to small-group sessions. One of the cases that shook students was depicted in a short documentary made in the early 1970s called *Please Let Me Die*. The title was disconcerting enough, the contents even more so. In it, a young fighter pilot and Vietnam veteran is first seen undergoing an obviously agonizing disinfectant bath with bleach over raw flesh. He is blind, partly deaf, and emaciated, though his condition was not the result of combat service. His ears and part of his face had been burned away, as had much of his hands. He didn't receive his wounds in the war, but rather in an accident with his dad while they were inspecting land that they were thinking of buying.

Leaking propane gas had settled in a creek bed and ignited while they tried to start their car. Donald (later known as Dax) Cowart, then a twenty-five-year-old active-duty Air Force reserve pilot, had been disfigured in a disaster in which his father died, while he was gravely injured. Yet another irony to the story is that Dax might not have survived the initial days and weeks had it not been for new medical therapies developed partly to address injuries incurred in Vietnam. But survive he did.

While Dax was undergoing the torments of his therapy (the film was so upsetting that a student fainted in one of these classes), including repeated surgeries and debriding of his dying skin followed by the bleach baths, he began to express a desire to die. Several months into his treatment, a psychiatrist, Dr. Robert White, was brought in to assess his competence to make such a decision. Much of the short film consists of the psychiatrist's interview of Dax in bed. Dax's reasoning seemed compelling: a formerly handsome young man trapped in a once virile but now seriously disfigured body with seemingly poor prospects for a satisfactory life, he was in relentless agony. In the film, Dr. White confessed that he was puzzled. Dax did not strike him as mentally ill, though he was clearly crying out as anyone would in such a predicament. Yet were he to be granted his wish to die, it was hard to see how that could work in practice. Even if someone gave him a gun, he couldn't use it because at that point he had no functional fingers. It would even be difficult for him to throw himself out of a window. If the treatment were stopped, the medical staff would not only have to witness his agonized dying, they would also have to decide whether they could or should aid in the process with pain medication that could itself be fatal.

Today we are much more familiar with issues of death and dying in the public arena and with issues created or exacerbated by advancing medical technologies, but in the 1970s this was a novel dilemma. Students found the case enormously upsetting, to say the least. Some sympathized with Dax's argument that care was being forced on him without his consent, but others focused on the fact that he could build a satisfactory life if he allowed his many devoted doctors and nurses to treat him. Still, why should he be forced to, and what realistic alternative was there? What about his ability to decide?

Like our beloved family members, Eva Brenner and Zerka Moreno, Dax's competence was being questioned, in his case not because of ageism or sexism but most likely out of uncertainty about the effects of the trauma and pain. Perhaps the trauma and pain were clouding his judgment, as some of his doctors believed. The challenge for those of us who used the film in the still somewhat experimental bioethics classes of the 1970s was in helping our students accept the very ambiguity of the situation. On its face, the principle of respect for autonomy supported Dax's decision, but the principle of nonmaleficence prohibited harming him. The bioethics principles set the terms of the dilemma but, as is often the case, didn't immediately resolve it. Still, no one wanted to walk out of the classroom with matters collectively unresolved. Emotions ran high even as the class period came to its inexorable end.

What struck the early bioethicists—who were drawn primarily from the fields of medicine, philosophy, and theology—was that their moral traditions and ideal theories of justice did them at best only limited good in the new world being made possible by medical technology. The principles were developed in light of bioethical issues, but they didn't provide a mechanical solution, let alone a certain one. A much longer documentary supervised by Dax himself some years later didn't make matters any easier. Called *Dax's Case*, the film featured interviews with various players in the drama, including his caregivers, the family lawyer, his best friend, and his mother, as well as Dax himself, now a lawyer in a Texas firm. Remarkably, no one changed their position from the views they had had years before. Dax continued to insist on his right to die even though the outcome was relatively favorable, a seeming paradox that utterly flummoxed many of the students. He even spoke of wanting to sue the hospital for care that he felt was forced on him at the same time as civil rights movements for others were flourishing. But not for grievously injured patients.

Over the next months and years, Dax did accept treatment though still under protest. Disfigured, blind, and partly deaf with only a few fingers remaining, he managed to complete law school, interrupted by problems with depression, and he married a couple of times. Dax read his poetry as a popular inspirational speaker and immersed himself in helping to train lawyers to be more sensitive to the needs of their clients and, through role-playing techniques, to be more appreciative of the total situation of a legal case. Dax is a frequent speaker on patients' rights. To this day, he believes he should not have been treated against his will and has expressed regret that he did not sue the hospital to refund his payments for imposing the unwanted treatment on him.

Not all the cases that attracted public attention in the first decade of modern bioethics involved high-technology medicine or serious disease, nor even physicians and patients. Some incidents called attention to shifting attitudes about the duties of health professionals to the public. One that undergraduates found especially disturbing, and that continues to roil debates about the duties of health care professionals, was the case of a University of California, Berkeley, student named Tatiana Tarasoff. In 1969 Tarasoff was murdered by a mentally ill young man, Prosenjit Poddar, who was upset that she had rejected his wish for a romantic relationship. Poddar had been seen by a psychologist at a University of California clinic and told him of his plan to murder Tarasoff. At the request of his campus psychologist, Poddar was briefly detained by campus police but then released. Bizarrely, Poddar lived with Tarasoff's brother before he stabbed her to death. Neither Tarasoff nor her parents were warned of the threat.

In their lawsuit, Tarasoff's parents argued that the psychologist and the university had a duty to warn them and their daughter of Poddar's detailed statements of his murderous intent. In 1976 the California Supreme Court agreed that a health care professional's duty of confidentiality could be trumped by knowledge of a danger to the public. The court held that "protection of the confidential character of patient-psychotherapist communications must yield to the extent to which disclosure is essential to avert danger to others." A dissenting opinion argued that such a significant limit on confidentiality of patient communications with mental health professionals would undermine their very practice. In 2013 the president of the American Psychological Association denounced the Tarasoff decision as "bad law, bad social science, and bad social policy." Yet he, too, admitted exceptions to the duty of confidentiality as a last resort, if necessary to prevent one's patients from endangering others.

Even the most ancient ideas about medical ethics, such as the professional's duty of confidentiality, were publicly challenged in a new era that placed a greater emphasis on protecting both human life and human rights. While many U.S. states have since adopted Tarasoff statutes that limit the health care professional's duty of confidentiality for the sake of public safety, others have limited it through common law precedents, and still others recognize no legal limits. What should those ethical and legal limits be, and who should enforce them? The answers to these life-and-death questions remain highly controversial, and it has become not just health care professionals' or judges' but everybody's business to answer them.

BEYOND AN ACADEMIC DEBATE

While Dax's case was exposing early bioethics students to human suffering and Tarasoff's to the potential limits of confidentiality, a best-selling book, which seemed to come in the mid-1970s out of nowhere, was calling attention to animal suffering. A young Australian philosopher, Peter Singer first published *Animal Liberation* in 1975. Like many philosophers of his generation, Singer found purely theoretical approaches to philosophy insensitive to the struggles unfolding outside of academia, like the civil rights and the antiwar movements. He was among those who helped to revive an Anglo-American philosophical tradition that blended ethical analysis with an understanding of real-world problems in a way that illuminated the issues in question. For Singer, that issue was the ethical treatment of animals.

Movements for the humane treatment of animals long preceded Singer's book, which first appeared in Australia, but Singer put the issue in modern terms, referencing factory farms, the cosmetics industry, and at least raising questions about medical research involving animals. Remarkable for a book on philosophy, *Animal Liberation* became an essential read even among those of us who hadn't focused on that issue. It was also innovative in the way it both managed to present a well-established philosophical theory, utilitarianism, and apply it to graphic descriptions of presumably pain-inducing practices for often trivial reasons. For example, Singer explained that rabbits were commonly held in restraints when used to test the toxicity of cosmetics so that they couldn't wash away irritating substances. Various formulations could be compared to one another to see which were most harmful. Cringe-inducing examples like this brought a philosophical argument to public attention. It was unusual for a young philosopher to become so widely read and prominent, but with his unsparing arguments Singer touched a universal nerve. By the end of the 1970s, thanks in no small part to Singer, a course in the still nascent field of bioethics commonly included a session on animal rights, often represented by a selection of required reading from his book.

Singer posed the jarring question: Why is an animal's pain any less important than that of a human being? He popularized the term "speciesism," which he argued was akin to racism and no more defensible. Singer's deeply held utilitarian perspective built on British philosopher Jeremy Bentham's classic utilitarianism: the pain felt by any animal has to be taken as seriously as the equivalent level and amount of pain felt by a human being. Harking back to Bentham's famous (or infamous) position on natural rights as "nonsense on stilts," Singer's utilitarian philosophy rejected any foundational view of rights, whether animal or human. The practical effects of Singer's views were similar to older movements for the humane treatment of animals, such as those created in nineteenth-century England, but he grounded his views in a distinguished philosophical theory. Whether one agreed with his utilitarian approach or not (we do not), it was a good example of applying philosophical theories to real-world cases and reaching a conclusion that could lead to changes in social policy. In Singer's case, his book helped to fuel changes in the way the cosmetics industry tested its products as well as the ways that food animals like chickens and pigs are raised. *Animal Liberation* remains a striking example of the new generation of ethicists' influence on actual practices.

Another topic in those early bioethics courses was sometimes called "applied genetics." That topic fell into two categories: genetic testing and screening and manipulating DNA. In the case of genetic testing and screening, diseases like phenylketonuria (PKU), sickle cell, and Tay-Sachs could by the late 1960s be identified through blood tests. Huntington's disease testing followed, leading to agonizing decisions for prospective parents with a family history. Each condition stimulated its own debate. PKU can be managed with a limited, bland diet. Management is harder for sickle cell patients. Babies with Tay-Sachs live brief, difficult lives. And persons with Huntington's face a predictable, drawn-out period of decline and dementia. There was also a simmering debate with echoes from Aldous Huxley's (1932) *Brave New World*: Did the rapidly growing science of genetics portend an opportunity to prevent suffering and promote human flourishing or simply give us the illusion of control over our destiny?

PUBLIC BIOETHICS

The commonality of all these diverse cases—suffering made possible by modern medical care, limiting patient confidentiality, the ethical treatment of animals, and the fruits of applied genetics—exposed a world unprepared for the myriad choices foisted upon us by the ever-expanding scope and public prominence of biomedical treatments and technologies. The collision between long-established institutionalized practices and new, unavoidable choices seemed overwhelming.

The disquiet was palpable in the small seminar and conference rooms where newly minted bioethicists and their students met to discuss the issues raised by one fascinating and then novel case study after another. A clear signal that this was more than an academic debate was coming out of a few cutting-edge biology labs.

In the early 1970s, nearly twenty years after Watson and Crick decoded the genome, biologists figured out how to "recombine" DNA, potentially creating novel proteins that could express new traits in plants and animals. The technique was laborious, but scientists were excited that they were turning biology into an engineering field. Not everyone was so thrilled, especially in a few of the communities adjoining the campuses whose members feared that new and dangerous life forms could emanate from the proverbial science building down the street, a fear reflected in a 1950s B-movie called *The Blob* starring a young Steve McQueen, featuring an interstellar snot-like substance that proceeds to devour inhabitants of a small town.

Older science fiction was also a convenient reference point as one Harvard facility was called the "Frankenstein lab" by local activists. And there was reason for concern. No one could be sure that some manufactured organism might not escape from the lab and create a public health crisis, like a virus carrying a cancer gene to be studied in mouse cells. After a series of meetings and publications, the scientific community decided to take matters into its own hands and demonstrate their sense of public responsibility by declaring a voluntary moratorium on recombinant DNA research until the risks could be assessed. A 1975 conference at California's Asilomar Conference Center is a frequently cited milestone in the self-regulation of biology. Despite reservations among some scientists that the moratorium was an overreaction, it proved critical in controversies in which we participated decades later over how best to realize the many beneficial results of new technologies, while avoiding their greatest risks.

After Vietnam and Watergate, traditional ways of thinking in America were at risk, and so was the role of the stewards of those traditions. The emerging tensions, especially about ethics, could no longer be reliably referred to a clergy who spoke, even within each religion, with a much less unified voice. The relative liberalization of Vatican II under Pope John XXIII had exposed or perhaps created philosophical rifts among Roman Catholics. Many rabbis were aligning themselves with the African American civil rights movement. Among the first and most striking signs of modern political Islam appeared in the form of a revolution in Iran in 1979. At the same time, where once Americans thought of science in connection with the space program and "The Bomb," their thoughts increasingly turned toward new life-extending technologies and novel life-giving ones, like the first so-called test tube baby in 1978. Traditional religious sources of moral guidance had become much more pluralistic and divided in their perspectives while new ethical challenges—typically with no easy answers—were moving front and center in public life.

A Google Ngram search of millions of books shows a steep increase in the use of the term "ethicist" starting in 1975. The term first pops up in the 1850s, putters along for about eighty years, grows in the war-ridden 1940s, and settles down again until the rise of the new medicine, technology, and biology. The term "bioethicist" (more closely linked to health care than "ethicist") just began to gain traction in the early 1970s, coinciding with the whistleblower revelation of the U.S. Public Health Service's grossly unethical Tuskegee syphilis experiments, which we discuss in chapter 7. (To say that these experiments were grossly unethical became about as clear as any judgment can be, once their most basic facts were brought to public light.)

The decade of the 1980s saw an explosive growth in the use of the term "bioethicist," partly because of the media's need to identify these new experts who were commenting on dramatic medical cases. They were educated as doctors and nurses, philosophers and theologians, lawyers and other familiar professions, but none of these labels described their role as ethics analysts and commentators. Many people first heard the views of bioethicists in 1982, when a sixty-one-year-old dentist named Barney Clark received what all involved hoped would be the first permanent artificial heart. The quest for a mechanical pump for people with grave heart disease had been going on for decades, gaining impetus with the shortage of hearts for transplant.

At first, the public reaction to the experiment was largely positive, with Clark celebrated in the press as a new kind of medical pioneer along with his audacious surgeon, William DeVries. But then it became clear that the Jarvik-7 heart wasn't at all what many thought a permanently implanted artificial heart would be. Clark was tethered to a 350-pound machine that pumped air into his chest, causing severe discomfort and complications. By the time he died after a difficult 112 days that were covered by a fascinated media, bioethicists were among those who prominently raised red flags. As the historian Shelley McKellar observes:

> Most outspoken against the clinical use of artificial hearts, bioethicists contested issues of informed consent and patient autonomy, access and cost, quality of life and patient self-determination, and the overall criteria for success. A discernible shift in medical and lay discussions was evident; once focused predominantly on the feasibility of developing artificial hearts, they now extended to the desirability of such a clinically acceptable device (perfected or otherwise).

In the early 1990s, "bioethicist" gained even more ground as a new kind of public intellectual, paralleling the progress and ultimately the striking success of the international research project to map the whole human genome. That landmark was quickly followed by the headline-grabbing revelation in 1997 of the successful cloning of a mammal, famously named Dolly, from an adult cell the previous year. "Bioethicist" and "bioethics" continued to soar in use in the early twenty-first century, with ever-increasing national and international research, educational programs, dedicated organizations, and public interest in bioethical issues. The interest comes from diverse corners of society, from grassroots groups to the federal government, the pharmaceutical industry, the organized scientific community, and even the military and intelligence agencies.

Bioethics thus was born of heightened controversy and concerns over the changing doctor-patient relationship, blocked access to new medical discoveries and unaffordable health care, and the risk-laden consequences of scientific research on humans and animals. These issues percolated at the end of the last century and grew to heightened prominence in the last three decades. Bioethics gained greater prominence, we suspect not coincidentally, at the same time as the costs of health care were skyrocketing in the United States, and trust in moral and professional authorities, and in authority generally, was plummeting.

GRAPPLING WITH ABORTION

We trace our own consciousness of bioethical issues back to our childhoods: we learned not to lie or be deceptive, yet we discovered that doctors did so when it came to emotionally fraught matters of life and death. Over several decades, a major shift toward greater professional honesty with patients became broadly accepted and almost universally defended in the name of multiple values, including personal freedom, individual autonomy, well-earned communal trust, and respect for persons. These values were expressed along with demands for long-suppressed civil rights among African Americans, Native Americans, gays and lesbians, and women.

Yet the freedom of women to exercise control over their own bodies, consistent with the new bioethics of patient decision making and the women's rights struggle itself, has not taken root as it should. Before 1900, abortion was quite common and accepted at least until women could feel the first fetal movements, known as "quickening," usually around the fourth month of pregnancy. Leading up to the Supreme Court decision in the case of *Roe v. Wade* in 1973, abortion had become illegal in most states, although a minority had begun to relax their abortion restrictions. Beginning in the late 1960s, over a dozen states started allowing abortion in cases of rape, incest, danger to a woman's health, or a likely deformed fetus (or some combination of the above), and four states legalized abortion in almost all cases. In a few other states, courts struck down their abortion restrictions.

In 1969 an impoverished twenty-one-year-old Texas woman, Norma McCorvey, wanted to end her third pregnancy after having given up her first two children to adoption. Blocked by Texas law prohibiting abortion except to save the mother's life, Norma was represented by two Texas lawyers seeking a plaintiff to challenge anti-abortion laws, and she was identified as Jane Roe in court documents. The lawsuit was filed on behalf of Jane Roe and *all women* "who were or might become pregnant and want to consider all options" against Henry Wade, the district attorney of Dallas County, where McCorvey resided. The Texas district court declared the abortion ban illegal on grounds that it violated a constitutional right to privacy, but Wade defiantly stated that he'd continue to prosecute doctors who performed abortions.

The all-male U.S. Supreme Court that decided *Roe* three years later was keenly aware that the stakes in legalizing abortions were high not only for women seeking abortions but also for doctors who felt a professional obligation to provide them. In the seven-to-two Supreme Court decision in *Roe*, Justice Harry Blackmun wrote for the majority that on grounds of a constitutional right to privacy the choice to end a pregnancy in the first trimester was solely up to the woman and her physician; that between the first trimester and the point of fetal viability, abortion could be regulated in the interests of maternal health but not banned; and that after the point of fetal viability, the state could prohibit abortion unless the woman's health was in danger.

While major shifts in bioethical practices, such as the doctor-patient relationship, have become far less controversial over our lifetimes, the same has not been true of the legal empowerment of women to determine the fate of their pregnancy. Neither near-universal public acceptance nor near-universal scholarly defense of legalized abortion ensued. Since 1973, the trends of American public opinion have been volatile rather than moving steadily in the direction of identifying as "pro-choice" or "pro-life" on the issues of abortion. If (as we believe) women do and should have a constitutional right to make their own life decisions—and if that includes the right to end their pregnancy before the fetus is viable—then by the very nature of that right, it must not be subject to public opinion polls.

Still, it should not go without our wondering or worrying—since it is strikingly relevant to so many other contentious issues in bioethics, such as embryonic stem cell research (which we discuss in chapter 8)—why, unlike other shifts in bioethical practices, the legalization of abortion remains so very heated and divisive. Abortion clinics are criminally attacked and doctors performing abortions killed, while the number of abortion providers has dramatically declined from its high point in the early 1980s, and many added restrictions on abortion are controversially championed, some successfully and others not.

Why legalized abortion continues to be so publicly divisive is itself a divisive discussion. Some attribute the extreme divisiveness to the court's rendering too broad a decision, legalizing abortion nationwide, rather than more narrowly striking down the very restrictive Texas law and gradually moving toward more universal legalization as challenges to other differentially restrictive state laws mounted. Others cite evidence against attributing the polarization around abortion to *Roe v. Wade* and argue that in any case a narrow decision would have unjustifiably deprived women of a constitutional (and human) right that was already long overdue and desperately needed, especially by poor women, to make their own life decisions. (In states that banned abortion, women without financial resources were effectively unable to obtain a safe one.) Still others argue that abortion continues to have all the elements of a political "wedge" issue to enable the Democratic and Republican parties and candidates for public office to differentiate themselves as they compete in mobilizing and turning out the votes of their most avid base supporters, too often (to our minds) by demonizing their opponents. Backed by detailed evidence and arguments that fill many volumes, these explanations, as well as others, are all controversial, and some are not mutually exclusive. The contentiousness of the legal ethics and the democratic politics of abortion is, as social scientists say, overdetermined.

The ethical core of the abortion controversy hinges on the question of when the life of a human person with the full panoply of constitutional and human rights begins: "Pro-life advocates believe the fetus to be a human being—a person in the generic sense, with rights that should be constitutionally protected. . . . Pro-choice advocates believe the [embryo and] fetus to be only a potential constitutional person . . . [and] women [therefore] should have the liberty to decide whether to bear a child." In his writing for the court, Justice Blackmun noted that "We need not resolve the difficult questions of when life begins. When those trained in the respective disciplines of medicine, philosophy, and theology are unable to arrive at any consensus, the judiciary . . . is not in a position to speculate as to the answer." Rather than pretending to pull off the impossible of determining when human personhood begins, which would require either an ethical consensus or a certain conclusion on the part of the court that continues to elude the widest range of eminent scholars and the entire American public, Blackmun noted that "the unborn have never been recognized . . . as persons in the whole sense," and they are not protected by the right to life enumerated in the Fourteenth Amendment. The State, he argued, has a "compelling interest" in protecting potential human lives at their point of viability but not before.

Putting every other legal and political controversy over abortion aside, for an important moment: let's recognize just how unacceptable this (or any similar) decision to legalize abortion can be to those who firmly believe—*rightly or wrongly*—that embryos and fetuses are full-fledged human beings and should be treated as constitutional persons from conception (or any time shortly thereafter) onward. We say how unacceptable legalized abortion "can be" rather than "must be" to people who firmly believe the embryo or fetus to be a person:

that's because it's ethically plausible to believe that a fetus is a full-fledged human being but that women should have a right to decide for themselves whether to have an abortion. How's this ethically possible? Posing this question gives rise to animated and illuminating discussion in college classrooms and public forums. One strong but not definitive answer: because you can be "pro-life" in your own life but recognize that the basis of the pro-life position—like that of the pro-choice position—is reasonably contestable, that the status of the fetus is simply not provable beyond a reasonable doubt (whereas the status of women is). If there's a reasonable doubt, even if it's not a doubt that you yourself have, you may conclude that a woman's right to control her own life should prevail. In essence, this is the position of many people who morally oppose abortion but respect the right of women to make such a life-altering decision for themselves in most if not all circumstances.

But pro-life advocates generally do not accept the legalization of abortion in most circumstances, just as pro-choice advocates vehemently oppose reversing the abortion rights recognized by *Roe v. Wade*. Two years before *Roe v. Wade* was decided, the philosopher Roger Wertheimer captured what's rationally irresolvable about the ethical and ontological controversy at the core of the abortion controversy: "While the liberal stresses the differences between disparate stages [of fetal development from embryo to fetus to infant], the conservative stresses the resemblances between consecutive stages [from infant to fetus to embryo]." Wertheimer's conclusion helps to explain why the abortion debate is not resolvable by reason alone: reasoned argument "does not itself point in either direction: it is *we* who must point it, and *we* who are led by it. If you are led in one direction rather than the other, that is not because of logic, but because you respond in a certain way to certain facts [about the fetus]."

What the ongoing debate over abortion drives home—however we respond to certain (or uncertain) facts and values—is that bioethics, like the engaged intellectual traditions that help inform its practice, often finds itself immersed in political as well as ethical controversy.

And it is, in fact, everybody's business to weigh in on those controversies. As the life and liberty, life-and-death stakes of the abortion debate make clear, it's not only the business of lawyers and judges, philosophers and theologians, health care providers, employers, and politicians. Responsible teaching of bioethics in the classroom sets out these arguments and the reasoning behind them as well as noting how pervasive such strong disagreements are not only in the context of abortion itself, and not only in the clinical setting, but in the ethics of the life sciences more generally. The societal need for robust and respectful disagreement must also be conveyed. But how?

RESPECT ACROSS DIVIDES

In the earliest years of bioethics, trust across most social divides was stronger and political controversy more muted than in subsequent decades. Among the small early group of people interested in bioethics, disagreements about the moral status of the human embryo or fetus were no less vigorous and deeply held than they are now, but they tended to be both substantial and collegial. Recognizing the critical role of attitudes toward abortion in emerging bioethics, Hastings Center cofounder Daniel Callahan and his wife, the psychologist Sidney Callahan, wrote a book called *Abortion: Understanding Differences* about their deep disagreements on the issue (both Roman Catholics, he identifies as pro-choice and she as pro-life), and they engaged in a public dialogue. Over the years, Callahan has elaborated his own position as antiabortion and pro-choice, explaining that he is morally opposed to abortion on a personal level but he would not impose his moral stand on women who profoundly disagreed with him. He understands the most basic disagreement over the morality of abortion to be both profound and reasonable, as some philosophers like Wertheimer have explained and many people have experienced. For us, as for Callahan, the imposition of state power over a woman's body renders that option a violation of her basic liberty. To our knowledge neither of the

Callahans convinced the other to change their most basic pro-life or pro-choice positions.

Robust debate across rationally irresolvable divides is all the more valuable for the respect it demonstrates among those who may continue to fundamentally disagree with one another. That we can disagree robustly and respectfully is a great virtue, not only for the tolerance and respect for deep disagreement that it demonstrates but also because it's a basic building block of all democratic societies and educational institutions. Of course, most of us who disagree over abortion and other bioethical controversies aren't otherwise united by bonds of matrimony like the Callahans. As democratic citizens and lifelong learners, we fallible, fellow human beings therefore need to bridge greater chasms of corrosive mistrust to cultivate mutual respect, understanding, and agreement where possible across our ethical divides.

We can do this in multiple ways, beginning with listening to one another's stories and arguments about the issues that divide us with as open a mind and as generous a spirit as possible. Quite specifically, this means (among other things) not assuming, let alone claiming, that those with whom we disagree about abortion have bad motives (while we have admirable ones): they really just want to keep women in their place or they really have no reverence for human life. Impugning the motives of those with whom we disagree minimizes the potential for constructive cooperation across divides. By contrast, we can maximize that potential by economizing on our moral disagreements: we can try to find "significant points of convergence between one's own understandings and those of citizens whose positions, taken in their more comprehensive forms, we must reject." Pro-choice and pro-life advocates can join together, for example, in publicly supporting unwed mothers in need of child support. And, as the philosopher Judith Jarvis Thomson creatively argued, even someone who firmly believes that the fetus is a person can support abortion rights in the limited circumstances of rape and other involuntary pregnancies.

The issue of abortion continues to divide our society, often viciously so, lurking behind a wide range of debates we consider in this book, from end-of-life care to eugenics, embryonic stem cell research, and beyond. With the significant exceptions of a few high-profile individuals and those who are closely identified with faith traditions, bioethicists have generally not made abortion a centerpiece of their work. This may be because they find it to be so politically polarized that nuanced positions advancing the argument are largely unwelcome on all sides. Or it may be because the crux of the controversy—the moral status of the human embryo and fetus—is (as some philosophers argued decades ago) rationally irresolvable.

It may seem futile to stand up as we have for the value of searching for more common ground, economizing on our disagreements, and respecting those with whom we continue to disagree. But the fact that a majority of Americans express quite nuanced positions on abortion, positions that also change over time, suggests otherwise. To be sure, abortion continues to be a morally fraught controversy for just about everyone, from those who believe there is one clearly right answer that needs to be legally enforced to those who place great civic value on respecting reasonable disagreements in this divisive realm. We don't pretend to be able to resolve the controversy nor do we expect that others soon will. What we urge is more mutual understanding, toleration, and respect for one another across such rationally unresolvable divides.

Bioethics as a field has grown rapidly over the last decades of the twentieth century and the first decades of the twenty-first. At the same time, trust in almost all institutions and professionals has precipitously declined. Bioethical debates and deliberations involve more diverse individuals and groups, both nationally and globally, and the issues and the participants become more publicly prominent. The price to be paid for publicly confronting the widest range of bioethical controversies in the context of a polarized society is that civility and mutual respect across some inescapable divides cannot be taken for granted. These core civic values must be modeled, debated, and defended. Reason and tolerance remain among the Enlightenment's greatest gifts. Nowhere are they more important than in matters of life and liberty, birth and death.

The Enlightenment also framed a debate about the common good, an argument that has ancient origins. Rather than subordinating the individual to the power and will of the state as had been the view of many previous philosophers, John Locke argued that the role of the state is to protect its members' life, liberty, and property. Immanuel Kant considered all persons ends in themselves: they must never be treated *merely* as means to a collectivist end but always *also* as ends in themselves. If Kant's "categorical imperative" seems rather abstract, it famously is. Yet it also translates directly into respect for persons and a central ideal of modern clinical ethics: researchers must never treat patients as merely useful, expendable means to social ends even ones as important as discovering a powerful new vaccine or a cure for cancer. Informed consent has become a necessary Kantian condition of life science research and patient care. More of a collectivist, Jeremy Bentham argued that the common good—and the measure of right and wrong—should be seen as maximizing individual happiness. A government's duty is to serve its people by pursuing the greatest happiness of the greatest number.

What happens, though, when maximizing happiness or social welfare requires collective agreement to the state's providing fluoridated water to prevent tooth decay in children, or its requiring vaccinations to prevent infectious disease epidemics, or its deciding whether to create an opt-in or opt-out policy for organ donations? These kinds of decisions cannot realistically be unanimous among citizens for a morally pragmatic reason: a rule of unanimity empowers a few bad actors effectively to hold everyone else hostage to their refusal to consent. Democratic rights such as "no taxation without representation" are partly individual and partly collective in nature: they honor the right of every individual as an equal citizen to participate in collectively determining, often by majority vote, laws and policies that will be collectively binding. These democratic rights are themselves still a work in progress. They create some obvious tensions about the nature of the common good as against those individual rights that enable everyone to decide for herself—for example, whether to use fluoride or to get vaccinated. Since fluoride and vaccinations, to be effective, must be provided to children, it turns out that the individual right to decide for oneself cannot reasonably apply in these as in many other cases. Yet tensions persist between the realm of individual and collective decision making. And these tensions underlie still another bioethical controversy: armed with modern understanding of health and disease, what is the state's role in advancing the common good through public health policies and practices, and what are its ethical limits?

Three

THE PUBLIC'S
HEALTH

The ethics of public health are not as exotic as other bioethical issues raised by organ transplants, genetic screening and engineering, physician-assisted death, new reproductive technologies, stem cells, cloning, and brain science. Many "high-tech" topics seize the bioethical and public imagination as do the poignant end-of-life decisions confronting individuals and their families. Crises like the HIV/AIDS, Ebola, and Zika epidemics also grab headlines and intense public attention because they engender fear. Although in the modern world our thoughts may immediately turn to finding effective vaccines, they take years to develop and manufacture at scale. In the first instance, the hard work of containing an epidemic primarily involves lifesaving interventions, like community health education, that are far from headline grabbing.

Rather than focusing on high-tech and patient-based medicine, public health addresses entire populations. While more patient control over medical decisions has demanded an ethics of informed individual consent, this bioethical principle cannot guide population-based health care. Epidemics are neither prevented nor controlled by asking for every individual's consent to what's needed to protect an entire at-risk population. Instead, public health must focus on large-scale trade-offs between risks and benefits. Those trade-offs, including the critically important consequences of proactively preventing illness and disease in larger populations, are neglected at our peril. Over the last hundred years, clean water, improved nutrition, and population-wide vaccination programs have made some of the greatest differences in extending life spans and in improving the quality of life. Yet by any measure of cost-effectiveness in saving, extending, and improving lives, the United States underinvests in public health.

Among preventative medical interventions applied to large populations, the smallpox eradication campaign of the mid-twentieth century (1967–1979) was exemplary, estimated to have saved over 50 million lives, along with enormous nonlifesaving benefits, such as preventing blindness. In 1967 alone, smallpox affected 10–15 million people, killing over 2 million. Toward the end of the twentieth century (1993), the Chinese government launched a national program to eliminate the world's leading and most easily preventable cause of mental illness: iodine deficiency disorder (IDD). The Chinese accounted for 40 percent of the world's population at risk for IDD, and within five years, the incidence of IDD-caused diseases like goiter and cretinism dramatically declined. By every standard measurement that is used to assess the efficiency and effectiveness of health interventions— whether it is the alphabet soup of cost-benefit ratio (CBR), the return on investment (ROI), the cost of a quality-adjusted life year (QALY), or the cost of a disability-adjusted life year (DALY)—major public health interventions like these affirm Benjamin Franklin's maxim that "an ounce of prevention is worth a pound of cure."

High-technology medicine, partly because it is so complicated and expensive, has only recently begun to make great contributions to many lives. By contrast, safety improvements in the workplace, family planning services that help to reduce infant and maternal mortality, child nutrition programs, well-targeted educational campaigns on the risks of smoking, and the widespread creation of tobacco-free environments—to cite just a few public health initiatives—generally cost very little per life saved and improved. The overall lifesaving benefits of some public health initiatives are, without exaggeration, enormous. Tobacco control saved an estimated twenty-two million lives worldwide between 2008 and 2014.

COPING WITH CONTROVERSY

Many public health breakthroughs come with controversy, even when evidence abounds that they advance good health and save scarce resources, and even when no peer-reviewed article in a reputable scientific journal suggests otherwise. Water fluoridation, for example, dramatically decreases the incidence of dental caries in children. Dental caries (commonly called cavities or tooth decay), although rarely life-threatening, is often debilitating and it's still a major public health problem in most industrialized countries.

The dramatic decline in childhood caries found in a well-designed ten-year study in Newburgh, New York, paired with the "control" city of Kingston, convinced New York City's hesitant mayor Robert F. Wagner in 1957 to consider fluoridating the city's drinking water to help prevent tooth decay. (Three other paired cities in the United States and Canada demonstrated similarly positive results to New- burgh's.) Yet the mayor, known for his caution, didn't take a decisive stand and eight more years passed before New York introduced water fluoridation, in 1965. Some of our neighbors even considered water fluoridation a Communist plot to impose a toxic substance or forced medication on American citizens. A full-court press of advocates— including Benjamin Spock, the nation's most famous twentieth- century pediatrician, Eleanor Roosevelt, and Jackie Robinson, as well as a former governor of New York, labor leaders, hundreds of scien- tists, and mothers from all five boroughs—vigorously made the pub- lic case for fluoridation, and thus the issue was kept alive for many years. The evidence was solid that tooth decay in children decreased by about 60 percent in cities that added as little as one-part fluoride per million parts of drinking water, and at a tiny cost per person, leading an experienced Newburgh dentist who had witnessed the "before and after" results to comment in 1970, "Today, whenever I see a child with a mouthful of cavities, I know immediately he's [or she's] not from Newburgh."

A far more searing image than tooth decay that we took from

our childhoods was called the iron lung. That was the popular name given to the mechanical respirator used to help polio victims breathe when they couldn't do so on their own. Pictures in magazines of smiling children in iron lungs shocked a generation of children. They looked trapped in those long tubes, and in a way, they were. They could only see who was with them in mirrors mounted above their heads. During late summer, it wasn't unusual for parents to order their children to change out of wet clothes right away, lest they be stricken by polio. By then it was widely understood that President Franklin Roosevelt had been a victim, though he attempted to hide his paralysis. But if the president could get polio, anyone could. The development of the safe Salk polio vaccine at the University of Pittsburgh, however, freed countless parents and their children from the fear of the advancing epidemic. In an example of the confidence Americans had in their doctors and in the medical establishment, the highly publicized polio vaccination campaigns of the mid-1950s were to a large degree massive public health experiments. Many of them took place in public schools with local newspapers running pictures of children being injected—sometimes smiling for the camera, sometimes crying. Reassured that they were pioneers of public health, they were commonly rewarded with a lollipop.

Even without the lollipops, we are today very thankful to have had our polio vaccinations and our fluoridated water. Despite continuing controversies, evidence shows that polio vaccines pose no more than minimal risk to individuals and that over a population their aggregate benefits are exponentially greater than the overall risks. The most effective antidotes to the fears fueled by misinformation are proactive measures, including better and more universal science and ethics education at every level, and open, well-informed democratic deliberations about public health decisions that engage diverse individuals and communities. The ethics of public health demand clarity in the goals of any program, from education to vaccination, and efficacy in reaching those goals. Modern brain science, discussed in the epilogue, underscores that the most effective public health advertising often appeals overwhelmingly to our emotions rather than our reason, raising questions of whether, when, and why short-circuiting our conscious minds may be justified.

At every step in the process and progress of a public health program, evidence is critical, not only when a program is being considered but as it proceeds. Privacy considerations are also crucial because unlike so much medical decision making that is done at the individual level, public health programs are directed at population health. Disease reporting needs to be fair so that some groups aren't targeted simply based on race, ethnicity, or gender. Even health education, though it sounds benign, shouldn't be more burdensome to some than others. As the public health scholar Nancy Kass has pointed out, any public health proposal will be met with some dissent. In itself, that's not a reason to automatically abandon a program. But those dissents must be taken seriously, especially if they come from specific minorities or neighborhoods.

For the sake of both international stability and global justice, improvements in population health must also extend to low-income countries in a way that respects their people. Public health benefits of new genetic technologies include such potentially lifesaving measures as the ability to improve global nutrition through crops that survive despite climate change and the capacity to control the insect vectors of diseases like malaria and Zika. Although international political cooperation is irreplaceable in improving global public health, private philanthropy also plays an important role. Along with billions of dollars in other initiatives, the Bill and Melinda Gates Foundation is supporting a project to develop male mosquitoes designed with genes that limit the life span of their offspring.

THE VACCINE DEBATE

Among the most informative and troubling examples that drive home the importance of evidence in the progress of a public health program is understanding how autism became linked to childhood vaccines.

Many sad personal stories led some people, often concerned parents, to link autism in children to vaccines. The flood of such stories and their influence in turning large parts of the public against lifesaving vaccination programs—vocal opposition to proven vaccines continues to this day—were triggered by an article published in 1998 in the *Lancet*, a highly regarded, peer-reviewed general medical journal. The article was principally authored by a doctor, Andrew Wakefield, along with twelve coauthors. It linked the measles-mumps-rubella (MMR) vaccine to autism. It was based on only twelve cases, with no controls, and it did not explicitly claim to demonstrate a causal relation between the vaccine and autism. But Wakefield released a concurrent video suggesting just such a causal relationship. He also recommended suspending the MMR vaccine and replacing it with a single-antigen vaccine for which, it was only later discovered, he previously had filed a patent and was also being paid by lawyers seeking to sue MMR vaccine manufacturers. A press storm publicizing the study's findings followed its publication and release of the Wakefield video. Many parents panicked. Many refused to vaccinate their children. MMR vaccination rates plummeted.

A variety of needless public health tragedies surrounding vaccines continues because the evidence presented in that article was unreliable, based on parental recall of only twelve children. That would have been bad enough, but worse still, the evidence was fraudulent. Yet by the time its unreliability and fraudulence were discovered and publicized, the myth that vaccines cause autism and other neurological disorders had taken on a public life of its own, amply fueled by human-interest stories, no doubt aided by the prevalence of the internet.

The British journalist Brian Deer was able to uncover enough evidence to report that Wakefield had grossly falsified data about the children's conditions. By the time of these revelations, not only had damage been done, but it continues to this very day despite the fact that multiple carefully scrutinized studies find no connection whatsoever between vaccines and autism. But not all the personal stories made the false link between MMR and autism. Here's a snippet of one among countless human-interest stories that illustrates both their power and limitations, this one told in 2012 by Martine O'Callaghan, an Irish mother of an autistic child:

> A sunny afternoon in the Spring of 2009: a mother sits in a doctor's office, a chubby-cheeked one year old on her lap. The family doctor looks at his notes and asks Mam to confirm the birth date of the wriggling baby boy. Mam replied: "Happy Birthday little man!" [T]he doctor beams. "Now, just roll up his sleeve, we can let him get back to his birthday cake." Mam complies and the MMR [measles-mumps-rubella] vaccine is injected. . . . Ten days later: the tot wakes in the night, sobbing. His temperature is elevated. Mam administers paracetamol and kisses. Age two years and four months: the boy, centre of his Mammy and Daddy's world, is diagnosed as severely autistic. Coincidence. . . ?

O'Callaghan's answer to her pointed question "Coincidence?" is "YES!" (She leaves no doubt about the accuracy of her answer by adding details about the behavior of her beloved son that she observed prior to the doctor's visit.) She went public with the story about her son to help counter the many more stories that preceded hers claiming that the MMR vaccine triggers autism, stories that don't accept the possibility that coincidences happen all the time in life:

> The more I read, the more I realized the anti-vaccination groups were using my child's condition, which isn't a tragedy nor was it an event, to terrify parents into making poor health choices for their families and peddle their wares. Aside from causing the resurgence in diseases like pertussis [whooping cough] and measles, the anti-vaccination movement has done incredible harm to autistic people.

Human-interest stories are important to tell, and to tell in responsible ways, as O'Callaghan does, which obviously doesn't mean without passion. It does mean by considering reliable evidence when such evidence is available.

If we care about saving and improving the lives of children and adults alike, we must appreciate the contributions of ethically conducted and reported medical science to millions of people. These contributions increased exponentially over the past century, especially through antibiotics along with vaccinations that have eliminated or made rare diseases like those that terrified Americans a century ago, including polio, smallpox, measles, mumps, and diphtheria. It's also important to note that, with the exception of antibiotics that are individually prescribed, most of these contributions fall squarely into the broad category of public health: they required government programs that included not only public investments but also public mandates to vaccinate or otherwise cover large populations.

EVIDENCE FOR NUDGING

While some advances in public health, like vaccines, require the introduction and approval of a new health care mandate, other advances depend not on mandating anything new but rather on changing the default option or otherwise increasing the likelihood that we will choose the healthier among our options. When a city, for example, creates dedicated bicycle lanes and rent-a-bike kiosks, it nudges some of us toward bicycling more. If it doesn't want to do this, it would be foolish to initiate such programs, and only if bicycling is on balance safer and healthier than driving does it incentivize us in the right direction. When those in charge of school cafeterias arrange food to make it most likely that their students will choose the healthier of all available options, they are nudging students toward better health.

All of us can be nudged, rather than forced, to adopt healthier options. The general strategy is to make sure that the options easiest to choose are those most likely to produce greater health benefits. Nudging is a feature of what economist Richard Thaler and legal scholar Cass Sunstein call our "choice architecture." A group's choices can be arranged so that its members are nudged toward healthier options. That group's aggregate behavior is altered in a predictable way without anyone requiring or forbidding them to choose one or another among available options. Notice that all of these descriptions of nudging use the passive voice, begging a critically important question: Who does the nudging?

Consider a negative but all-too-common example of nudging, a form that we regularly encountered in our family lives long before Thaler and Sunstein began promoting the idea of nudging in positive, healthy directions. When our children were young, every supermarket within convenient shopping distance prominently (and, no doubt, strategically) placed shelves of sugary candy at the checkout counters to tempt our children, and us. While we adults could consciously avoid the candy aisles in the store, we couldn't conscientiously avoid the checkout counter. As much as it irritated us, we were nudged by supermarket owners—and often nagged by our children as well—to buy candy. Turns out that although much has changed over the decades (sugar-free gum is now common), sugar-loaded candy still prevails at checkout counters (and not only at supermarkets) and it exemplifies unhealthy choice architecture, which nudges us to buy what's unhealthy because it's hardest to resist. Thaler has popularized the term "sludging" for this kind of unhealthy nudging.

Nudging can and should be a positive instrument of public health. But for that to happen, we who are nudged need to publicly pressure "choice architects" to put *our* health above *their* profits. We also need to support good research and follow its findings to implement better ways of incentivizing healthy choices and making them more affordable. As Thaler and Sunstein put it:

It seems reasonable to say that people make good choices in contexts in which they have experience, good information, and prompt feedback—say, choosing among ice cream flavors. People know whether they like chocolate, vanilla, coffee, licorice, or something else. They do less well in contexts in which they are inexperienced and poorly informed, and in which feedback is slow or infrequent—say, in choosing between fruit and ice cream (where the long-term effects are slow and feedback is poor) or in choosing among medical treatments or investment options. If you are given fifty prescription drug plans, with multiple and varying features, you might benefit from a little help. So long as people are not choosing perfectly, some changes in the choice architecture could make their lives go better (as judged by their own preferences, not those of some bureaucrat).

Thaler and Sunstein's parenthetical consideration is key, and it cannot be taken for granted. Nudging is good policy if (but only if!) it will make our lives go better by our own collective, democratically accountable preferences—not the government bureaucrat's, the advertising executive's, or the supermarket owner's.

Nudging has potentially broad-ranging applications to public health and to health care more generally. Some experiments test different ways of nudging people who want to stop smoking, exercise more, or lose weight. What's generally more effective: telling us that we will lose something if we fail or telling us that we will be rewarded (with something of comparable value) if we succeed? It turns out that we humans are more sensitive to loss than to gain, and significantly so (by a factor of about two to one). We are more likely to stick to a healthy regimen when we know that we'll lose money if we fail rather than when we know we'll be rewarded (with the same amount) if we succeed. These empirical findings raise an important ethical issue for the design of nudging "choice architecture": How is it possible to effectively incentivize but not penalize those individuals who cannot afford to lose money but who want to lose weight, exercise, or stop smoking just as much as anyone else? Informed participants may be given the option of receiving money up front—as a reward for future success—knowing that they may keep it only if they stick to their chosen healthy regimen. One study found that people were most likely to exercise, for example, with such an up-front payment plan, compared to reward-as-you-succeed or old-fashioned encouragement options.

In chapter 6, we consider the scarcity of organ donations for those whose lives depend on them, and we return to the ethics and practicality of nudging, not to improve our own health but to save other people's lives. Would you support a proposal that your government make consent to organ donation the default option when you are asked on, say, a driver's license application whether you choose to be an organ donor upon your death? A choice architecture that depends on opting out of organ donation instead of opting in would be a nudge in a certain direction, one that has the potential for saving many lives. This is just one among many possibilities of nudging for public and private health goals. Research findings are shedding more light on what works for worthy goals, and as a result, we now face collective ethical decisions about how to use nudging as a means for saving lives that may be our own.

Nudging has been both criticized and praised as paternalistic. Its advocates defend its "libertarian paternalism" for helping people to help themselves without forcing them to do so. Critics are concerned that its paternalism intentionally encourages people to accept benefits that they themselves haven't carefully and consciously chosen, and often haven't had time to think about, even if those benefits are in their best interests. (Advocates also oppose people being nudged against their best interests.) Although any of us could someday need an organ, some people object to nudging, especially if it comes from government and elite "experts" (whose track records of acting in the public interest are far from pristine). Then what should we do about all the nudging that's controlled by collective, not individual, interests? Companies that manufacture all those sugary sweets can be powerful opponents of removing them from checkout counters, though the result is that they are then the ones doing the nudging to protect their financial interests.

When in 2016 Philadelphia became the first major American city to pass a soda tax, Mayor Jim Kenney notably championed the tax not only (or even mainly) for public health but importantly to also fund public schools, parks, and libraries. The American Beverage Association immediately challenged the tax in court as unconstitutional, having spent millions opposing its passage. The largest contributor to a multi-million-dollar media campaign defending Philadelphia's soda tax was former New York City mayor Michael Bloomberg, whose ban on the sale of jumbo sodas in NYC had been struck down as unconstitutional just two years earlier. "Obesity and poverty," Bloomberg noted, "are both intractable national problems. No policy takes more direct aim at both than Philadelphia's tax on sugary drinks." The Pennsylvania Supreme Court upheld the soda tax in 2018, ending the court battle, but as the "Ax the Bev Tax" coalition declared, its war to sway public opinion and lobby city officials against the tax will continue. The soda tax campaign and controversy exemplify the fact that we all have a stake in addressing whether and how to nudge and be nudged.

Unlike informed consent for individuals, which upholds every patient's "right to be wrong" about what is good for them, nudging strives to advance population-wide benefits. So in order to avoid affronts to the self-respect and dignity of individuals, what's needed is the moral equivalent of informed, collective consent for a nudge campaign. That's not an easy task but neither is achieving informed consent by individuals to complex health care options. Much more attention has been paid—including by bioethicists and public officials—to the conditions of informed *individual* consent. For the sake of public health, we would do well to direct more attention to the conditions of informed *collective* consent. For a start, informed collective consent will include maximal feasible transparency of available alternatives. It will need to tell us how each alternative is likely to work. Nudging programs will need extensive public input as well as careful consideration of a reasonable set of exceptions that don't gravely undermine the larger goal of advancing public well-being.

MENTAL ILLNESS AND PUBLIC HEALTH

If public health is too little appreciated as a source of societal well-being, mental health care is too often entirely neglected. Mental illness is the costliest condition in the United States, with annual costs of at least $467 billion in 2012, and that number cannot begin to capture the human suffering for patients and their families. And for the seriously mentally ill, the situation has only gotten worse. In the words of one historian of mental illness, "those who suffer from serious psychoses make up one of the few segments of our societies whose life expectancy has declined over the past quarter of a century." Whether it's because of the social stigma that still attaches to mental illness or the frustrations involved in effective treatment or simply due to the expense of intensive interventions, the United States has never implemented a public mental health program that comes close to meeting ethical policy standards. Going back to the 1960s, there were strong arguments for "deinstitutionalizing" people with mental illness from hospitals that had grown too large, were under-funded, and sometimes downright chaotic. Advocates for closing the old asylums noted the availability of new antipsychotic medications. They also cited alleged violations of human rights and the prospect of shifting precious resources away from crowded institutions toward community-based treatment modalities.

During the Kennedy, Johnson, and Nixon administrations, plans were developed to create a network of community mental health centers for patients who required continued supervision. For various reasons, however, those centers never fully materialized. One result of that policy failure is a homeless population that now includes hundreds of thousands of people with serious mental illness. Another result is the increase of the U.S. prison population. Though estimates vary, as many as half of all incarcerated individuals have a mental illness and about one-quarter have a serious mental illness, such as schizophrenia. Experts have observed that prisons and jails have become the new psychiatric hospitals, and it goes without saying that they are extremely inappropriate settings to provide the care needed.

Besides the evident failures of deinstitutionalization, the prevalent mental health problems among children and adolescents have become the focus of considerable public attention in the second decade of this century. Anxiety, depression, and eating disorders, as well as epidemics of suicidality and abuse of opioids have renewed focus on mental illness as a public health problem. But as of today, the governmental response has been anything but robust. Mental illness is still stigmatized despite progress in public understanding, and its treatment and prevention remain desperately underfunded. This is true not only on an absolute basis of what would be "ideal," but also on a relative basis compared to other less debilitating, less treatable, and less prevalent illnesses.

Unlike the early years when the focus was on experiments with people with mental illness, bioethics has more recently concentrated on reforms in the mental health system as a whole with the potential to address the health care needs of millions more people. Especially with regard to the seriously mentally ill, bioethicist Dominic Sisti has addressed a wide range of ethical challenges: How should the right to liberty be balanced against the danger someone poses to oneself or others? Should people who don't object to treatment be "nudged" into accepting hospitalization? If long-term care "asylums" should be brought back for the most severe cases, what protections must be built into a system of long-term care? With so few long-term psychiatric beds left in the system, what can be done to ensure that mental health needs are given their due alongside other medical needs? Meanwhile, many severely mentally ill people are housed in jails and prisons, raising one of the most urgent questions of all: What obligations does society have to provide resources to people with severe mental illness who are in correctional settings and to aid the personnel who have not been trained to deal with those challenges?

The seriously mentally ill may have difficulty sustaining relationships. They are often without family members or friends who can

advocate for them. Few vote, attend town hall meetings, or participate in civic organizations. About them bioethics asks the most challenging moral questions that will appear in other contexts as well:
What is owed to those who have no voice or who have lost it? Who
decides for them? And who cares for them?

Someday, they will be us.

Part Two

MATTERS
OF LIFE
AND
DEATH

Four

UNEASY
DEATHS

How do we want to die? The question is both strange and obvious. It does not ask us "whether" but "how." The two questions are yoked together in the human psyche. Our primordial will to live and anticipatory anxiety over dying easily overwhelm our ability to address how we want to die. The irony of course is that we can exercise some degree of control only over how, not whether, we will die. Yet we often find it hard to move beyond the shadow question that might somehow promise eternal life to the practical one that asks us to consider how we want to approach the circumstances of our death. When we do thoughtfully probe ourselves and our loved ones about how we want to die, we discover that our preferences differ, sometimes quite unexpectedly.

What is virtually universal about the "preferred" circumstance of death is its association with ripe age. While what's considered ripe varies over time and across contexts, for every culture, premature death is deeply troubling and somehow seemingly unnatural. When a young person on the cusp of life faces a drawn-out, predictable dying process that deprives her of the future of love, family, and accomplishment that will always be just beyond her grasp, the reality can be too much to bear. Especially in an era that celebrates science and technology, when biomedical breakthroughs seem always just around the corner, it can be all the more agonizing to accept our limitations and constrained choices. This is true not only when further treatment proves unable to restore or even maintain a patient's health, but doubly so when a terminally ill patient seeks a medical intervention to hasten death.

BRITTANY'S CHOICE

These elements all came into focus in the case of Brittany Maynard, a twenty-nine-year-old University of California graduate with a remarkable passion for travel and giving to others less advantaged than herself, which propelled her to teaching in orphanages in Nepal. In 2014 she was diagnosed with a form of brain cancer. After two brain surgeries, the cancer returned a few months later in a more aggressive form. Her prognosis was terminal, with a most devastating form of brain cancer (glioblastoma multiforme) and about six months to live. She and her family were advised about the best available treatments, which included full brain radiation, to extend her life as long as possible but with severe side effects. She seriously considered passing away in hospice care, but reflected:

> My quality of life, as I knew it, would be gone . . . and the recommended treatments would have destroyed the time I had left. . . . Even with palliative medication, I could develop potentially morphine-resistant pain and suffer personality changes and verbal, cognitive and motor loss of virtually any kind.

Maynard moved from California and became a resident of Oregon so that she could satisfy all the legal requirements to be prescribed a life-ending drug by her doctor. During her last months, she became an articulate and appealing advocate for physician-assisted death, featuring in newspaper articles and television interviews. Her message, as thoughtful as it is poignant, calls upon us to share it:

I would not tell anyone else that he or she should choose death with dignity. My question is: . . . Why should anyone have the right to make that choice for me? . . .

I plan to celebrate my husband's birthday on October 26 with him and our family. Unless my condition improves dramatically, I will look to pass soon thereafter.

I hope for the sake of my fellow American citizens that I'll never meet that this option is available to you. If you ever find yourself walking a mile in my shoes, I hope that you would at least be given the same choice and that no one tries to take it from you.

When my suffering becomes too great, I can say to all those I love, "I love you; come be by my side, and come say goodbye as I pass into whatever's next." I will die upstairs in my bedroom with my husband, mother, stepfather and best friend by my side and pass peacefully. I can't imagine trying to rob anyone else of that choice.

That she was supported by her husband of less than two years, who also appeared on television, only seemed to add to the public agony.

Maynard's youth and vigorous advocacy marked a turning point in the modern right-to-die debate that had gathered steam over several decades. When the governor of California signed that state's physician-assisted death bill into law, it was partly under the influence of her case, a sign that the politics of the issue had changed, if not the ethics. Americans have long been accustomed to tragic news reports of older people faced with intractable illness, couples that died together, or even those in which one took the life of a beloved partner to spare the other from further suffering. In her evident vitality, Brittany Maynard shook these familiar frameworks. She also represented a newer attitude toward the medical system, a generation more prepared to take its assets into its own hands, even to demand that opportunity in the face of strong opposition from much of the medical community. In this way, her case resonates with the "right to try" movement for experimental medication that we discuss in chapter 5. But while the "death with dignity" movement also advocates for greater patient autonomy, unlike the "right to try" untested treatments, it fully accepts the scientific expertise of doctors to prescribe effective ones. What it challenges is their moral authority or the state's to overrule a patient's own informed consideration of what it means to die with dignity.

The Brittany Maynard case was a landmark in the movement for physician-assisted death. Whether for good or ill depends on where you stand on this case, but in any event it can't be fully understood or evaluated on its own. Among terminally ill patients, those who employ such medical means to hasten their death under "death with dignity" laws are a small minority. Vastly more Americans annually received hospice care, designed to provide more pain-free, compassionate, comforting, and dignified care to terminally ill patients (and to attend to their families as well). In order to comply with Oregon's "death with dignity" law, Maynard had to be informed about hospice care. Yet vast numbers of her fellow Americans who could benefit from hospice or other palliative care are not informed about it or cannot access or afford it.

Modern medicine gives doctors an ever-increasing capacity to order up tests and procedures, while American health care generally enables them to make more money by doing so. Yet hospice (or other palliative care) has demonstrated enormous potential for improving end-of-life care for millions more people, even if it cannot credibly promise to provide everyone a death with dignity and without needless pain and suffering. We'll return to examine its role in cultivating a common ethical ground amid ongoing legal and political controversies surrounding end-of-life care in America.

Legal and political systems don't necessarily settle ethical questions, and questions as profound as how much control we should have over our own deaths must be set against their cultural and historical background. An important preliminary step is to think broadly about the way death and dying are experienced as part of a life and not as discrete occurrences.

A MEANINGFUL DEATH

In 1965 the philosopher Simone de Beauvoir published a searing memoir of her mother's death from cancer. Their relationship had long been strained, partly by her mother's insistence that de Beauvoir renounce her atheism and return to God. As her mother reaches the end, the account is hard to read:

> Then suddenly she cried out, a burning pain in her left buttock. It was not at all surprising. Her flayed body was bathing in the uric acid that oozed from her skin. . . . All tense on the edge of shrieking, she moaned, "It burns, it's awful; I can't stand it. I can't bear it any longer." And half sobbing, "I'm so utterly miserable," in that child's voice that pierced me to the heart. How completely alone she was! I touched her, I talked to her; but it was impossible to enter into her suffering. . . . Nothing on earth could possibly justify these moments of pointless torment.

Then came a sudden spasm. As she cried that she couldn't breathe, de Beauvoir's mother lapsed into a coma and died soon thereafter. Later de Beauvoir reflected with her mother's nurse on the travails of her suffering. " 'But, Madame,' replied the nurse, 'I assure you it was a very easy death.' " As readers, we might be shocked at the nurse's casual attitude about what could remind us of the trials of Job, but de Beauvoir derives a larger point:

> For indeed, comparatively speaking, her death was an easy one. . . . I thought of all those who have no one to make that appeal to: what agony it must be to feel oneself a defenceless thing, utterly at the mercy of indifferent doctors and over-worked nurses. No hand on the forehead when terror seizes them; no

sedative as soon as pain begins to tear them. . . . She had a very easy death; an upper-class death.

To die in relative comfort surrounded by caring hands is for most of us the very least that we would want for ourselves and those we love. But still, de Beauvoir is unwilling to attribute greater meaning to her mother's dying process, or to that of anyone. That is not the usual philosophical or religious reaction to death. Plato ascribes meaning to the death of his beloved teacher Socrates, who refused to accept the opportunity to escape his death sentence, as was widely expected, on the grounds that to do so would entail a contradiction. Having chosen to live in Athens, fighting in its wars and raising his children in its domain, Socrates argued that he could not flout the state's ability to enforce its laws simply because he disagreed with a single judgment it had made. Calmly and cheerfully, as his friends wept and wailed, he drank the hemlock. The example of Socrates' death as a meaningful, conscientious, and even heroic event has had enormous influence in both secular and religious traditions.

These and other philosophers' accounts of the deaths of those close to them reflect the elemental human struggle to make sense of death or to abandon the notion that death can have sense. Yet this timeless dilemma tells us almost nothing about how human beings have actually died, and in fact our knowledge of the history of death before the last couple of hundred years is extremely thin. Great traumatic events like wars, plagues, and famine are recorded, but the deaths of ordinary people in ordinary times mainly involve a lot of guesswork. What we can say is that until very recently people died at home with little or no effective medical intervention. The physician's role was mainly to comfort and perhaps provide a prognosis. "Therapies" were often called by such terms as "heroic" not because they were rare but because they were so extreme. More often, the end came rapidly as compared to modern hospital death and certainly without the data from monitoring devices and laboratory tests that often provide no more than an illusory sense of control.

In a basic physiological sense all death happens the same way, when the brain is deprived of oxygen. Over the last sixty years, this recognition helped drive the development of a series of treatments grouped under the heading of "Advanced Cardiac Life Support." One of these treatments, cardiopulmonary resuscitation (CPR), has been at the forefront of medical ethics debates as doctors and institutions, with a large dose of legal liability, have tried to decide when CPR should be tried and how far it should go. Do-not-resuscitate (DNR) orders are now commonly recorded for patients who don't want CPR. The origin of DNR orders is closely tied to the death-and-dying debate in bioethics. Like many other medical technologies in the 1960s, CPR migrated from a drastic measure used in extreme situations to extend life to a nearly routine assumption for dying patients. Unfortunately, the results of resuscitation sometimes left patients alive but gravely impaired. In 1974 the American Heart Association recommended that doctors get consent for CPR, but practices still varied widely. Some hospitals were very aggressive, resuscitating patients many times, while others used codes, like purple dots, in medical charts to denote a DNR.

In bioethics as in life, there are some very strange coincidences. In 1975, just a year after the American Heart Association's recommendations, a twenty-one-year-old woman named Karen Ann Quinlan collapsed at a party at a bar near her home in New Jersey. She hadn't eaten for a couple of days and at the party she drank alcohol and used a sedative that was then a popular recreational drug. Feeling faint, she was taken home by friends, where she stopped breathing. She was given mouth-to-mouth resuscitation but she never regained consciousness, lapsing into a coma and then into a persistent vegetative state (PVS) due to significant brain damage, but she was not brain dead. This story is so critical to relate because it came to the fore as one of the most famous and polarizing bioethical issues of the 1970s and 1980s. Continuously covered by the media, her name resonated in popular culture, so much so that she became the subject of cruel jokes.

As it turned out, Quinlan was placed on a ventilator to ensure that she would breathe, and she received tube feeding. With spiritual advice and support from their pastor, her parents argued that the Catholic church's doctrine that "extraordinary means" to sustain life were not ethically required applied to her ventilator. The Quinlans fully expected that the hospital doctors would agree to remove their daughter from the respirator. When they refused, the Quinlans petitioned the state court to let their daughter die "with grace and dignity" by permitting its removal. This was a first for any American court to decide, and the heated courtroom drama included an attorney for the doctors arguing that a decision in favor of the parents' petition would be "like turning on the gas chamber."

The Quinlans lost that court case but they ultimately won on appeal against the State of New Jersey. The New Jersey Supreme Court issued a unanimous decision in support of a right to privacy concerning decisions about life-sustaining treatment. Karen Quinlan's ventilator was removed but she continued to breathe, unassisted, for nine years. She weighed sixty-five pounds when she died in 1985. The decision of Quinlan's parents not to remove the feeding tubes (on grounds that they were not causing her pain) left open a question to be addressed in later cases.

CLINICAL ETHICS

Though CPR was not the main issue in the Quinlan case, her story drew national attention to the range of issues around death and dying at a time when society was still adjusting to modern medical technologies. The physician and science writer Lewis Thomas coined the term "halfway technologies" that could maintain life but not return people anywhere close to their previous quality of life. In popular culture, the 1981 film *Whose Life Is It Anyway?*, starring the Canadian actor Richard Dreyfuss, told the story of a sculptor who had been left without the use of his arms and legs after an accident and asked to be helped to die. Somewhat ironically, as the first famous death-and-dying case, it was Karen Quinlan, a woman who could not ask herself for treatments to be stopped, whose situation propelled a bioethics conversation that dominated the 1980s.

A key moment in that conversation took place in 1983, with the publication of a presidential ethics commission's report called *Deciding to Forego Life-Sustaining Treatment*. The Dreyfuss film, the real-life Quinlan case, and all the related issues were no doubt very much on the commission's mind—and that of an interested American public—as it pondered the ethics of stopping a treatment that was keeping a patient alive at the request of that patient or her legal proxy. That a competent adult had the moral and legal right to decline treatment was less in question than what could be done if life sustaining had already begun, perhaps while the patient was unable to give consent. Would a physician who withdrew such treatment be responsible for the patient's death, even if that was clearly what the patient (or her proxy) wanted and understood that the likely result would be her death? The commission's conclusion was unequivocal: a patient does not need to have unwanted treatment continued any more than she would have to accept that treatment if it had not been started.

The commission argued that stopping a treatment is no more morally problematic than not starting treatment in the first place. And it went one counterintuitive step further. While most people find it psychologically harder to withdraw life support than to not start it in the first place, the practical ethics for professional health care providers, the commission reasoned, cuts in precisely the opposite direction. Whether an approved treatment will improve the condition of a particular patient before it has been tried is often highly uncertain. Consequently, professionals responsible for a patient's care may have *greater* justification—based on having *better* evidence—to withdraw an approved treatment once it's been found ineffective in a particular case than they have to withhold it before knowing its efficacy in that case. Erecting a higher hurdle for stopping treatment than for starting it, just because a patient's death may be foreseeably imminent, creates a perverse incentive for doctors to err on the side of not providing some patients with potentially lifesaving treatments.

The commission's report effectively collapsed any inherent ethical difference between a doctor withholding life-sustaining treatment and withdrawing it, even in the case of supporting breathing with a ventilator. This conclusion was unassailable as a matter of logic, but not as a matter of psychology. The commission recognized that, for a doctor, extubating a patient or "pulling the plug" typically *feels* very different from not starting the patient on the therapy in the first place. Yet in other less immediate life-and-death situations, the psychological burden generally is reversed. Consider a sober decision by a patient with a terminal cancer and her doctor to stop chemotherapy: this might well feel like less of a psychological burden for the doctor than not starting chemotherapy in the first place.

The commission carefully argued that psychological reactions shouldn't necessarily drive ethical conclusions. Those reactions are no less important; indeed, they are all the more important to understand. Although the commission's major conclusion—withdrawing medical treatment is not inherently more morally problematic than withholding it—remains controversial, it represents rapidly shifting attitudes among both the medical community and the public in the context of technological innovations of the 1960s and 1970s, high-profile legal cases, and evolving hospital-patient and doctor-patient relations.

The legal system is a poor substitute for achieving ethical consensus. In the hopes of avoiding cases like that of Karen Ann Quinlan in the 1970s, many hospitals created ethics committees to help resolve medical and ethical disagreements before they enter the legal system. These committees are often composed of doctors, nurses, social workers, and a community representative. Sometimes they are available to conduct emergency consultations. An ethics consultation can provide a nonthreatening setting in which disagreements can be aired and communication improved. As the historian David Rothman observed in his aptly titled history of bioethics *Strangers at the Bedside*, ethics committees are another example of the transformation of health care in America: medical ethics could no longer be the sole province of the physician in charge of a case.

ETHICAL CASUISTRY

Decisions about death are about as morally controversial as any, and how best to evaluate those decisions is no less so. As we noted earlier, amid the social upheavals of the 1960s and 1970s, many philosophers became committed to showing how rigorous moral reasoning is relevant to real-world problems. In their influential textbook, bioethicists Tom Beauchamp and James Childress set out to look for midlevel principles that are accepted by a wide range of grand moral traditions and are relevant to reasoning through actual bioethical dilemmas, like what are the limits on what can be done to people in potentially important research. They arrived at a set of four principles that they argued could be found in different ways in many philosophical and theological traditions: respect for autonomy, beneficence, nonmaleficence, and justice.

Some critics of what is sometimes called "principlism" noted that principles like autonomy and beneficence often lead to competing conclusions or no conclusion at all. Respecting the autonomy of a few people in research who are unable to consent, for example, competes with the beneficence of developing a lifesaving medication that could benefit countless patients. Regarding end-of-life care, even if we consider the ethical treatment of only a single patient, beneficence may conflict with autonomy or simply be indeterminate in commonplace cases where the patient is terminally ill, apparently suffering, not competent to decide, and lacking any advance directive. What then does an ethical health care provider or proxy decision maker do? Surely not simply note that these principles don't dictate a decision and say or do nothing more. In cases of conflict or indeterminacy, Beauchamp and Childress argued for balancing and specifying the principles. Critics, however, claimed that arguing from principles alone neglected a long-standing way of deciding challenging cases that is inherently more practical and no less moral. As well, often one can't simply infer the most beneficent action from the known facts of a case. Would Dax have been better off dead than he was by continuing to live?

Considering the limits of principlism, two prominent critics, Albert Jonsen and Stephen Toulmin, called for a renewal of interest in a case-based method of reasoning called casuistry, typically used in the common law and in theology. Put simply, casuistry involves assessing a line of cases about the same core problem, agreeing at one extreme on cases that are admirable and at the other extreme on those that are wholly unacceptable in how they were handled. In human experiments, at one end would be an important low-risk study with a fully informed and competent adult who could benefit, while the kinds of experiments done in the Nazi concentration camps would be at the other. In between, there would be all sorts of variations in detail that call for further detailed deliberation.

Consider a core question of medical ethics: How much knowledge and understanding does it take to be sufficiently informed to consent to an experimental treatment? Instead of trying to answer this question in all its generality, casuistry begins by posing specific questions of actual cases. Drawing upon the best precedents and the facts of this case, what does this particular patient need to know and why? Contextual reasoning plus analogies to well-established cases help to determine where a new case falls. Casuists worry that when we begin with general principles and proceed deductively to arrive at answers to particular cases, the principles become slogans, convey false certainty, and at the extreme support fanaticism.

Understanding actual cases is essential to bioethics as an enterprise of practical deliberation, but case analysis itself is incomplete without some guiding principles or their equivalent (for example, "rules of thumb" informed by principles). The more casuistry becomes its own independent method of inquiry, divorced from principles, the more readily it will be abused. The worst abuse amounts to reasoning from analogy or intuition to rationalize the unethical, which is the flip side of invoking principles to convey false certainty or defend fanatical intransigence. Imagine, for example, a "best case" of racial segregation as against a "worst case." Without a principle of human moral equality, we may be caught in an inherently immoral range of cases.

Short of making the immoral seem moral, the very word "casuistry" has come to stand for cleverly employing the most minuscule distinctions and losing sight of what's most morally important. In the case of human experiments, for example, we would never want to lose sight of respect for the autonomy or informed consent of individuals, while also recognizing the beneficent role of ethical experiments in finding new cures for fatal illnesses. (And that's just for a start.) When casuistry rejects the use of principles, it fails to recognize that they serve as important guides to our ethical understanding and are no less contextual than common maxims like "do unto others" or "walk a mile in their shoes." Using only analogies and examples without guiding principles can be sloppy at best and biased at worst. Ethical casuistry is a method of reasoning from paradigms and analogies that draws upon moral principles. We've found it an illuminating way to teach bioethics and a productive way to practice it.

Consider, for example, the contrasting Quinlan-era case of Joseph Saikewicz, who was sixty-seven years old when he was diagnosed with leukemia in 1976. Chemotherapy would have given him a 30–50 percent chance of remission for about a year. A resident of state institutions for nearly his whole life, Saikewicz had a severe intellectual disability with an IQ said to be about ten. He had no contact with family, so a probate court was responsible for his medical decision making. The court decided that treatment would not be in his best interests because it would have involved burdens he could not have understood for too little benefit to him. Chemotherapy was withheld, and he died a few months after his diagnosis.

Unlike the other cases we are discussing, Saikewicz not only was unable to decide for himself; he never had the capacity or therefore the opportunity to develop and express his own values and preferences. Because Saikewicz could not exercise autonomy, the probate court implicitly used the principle of beneficence in deciding on his behalf. In terms of ethical casuistry, if the paradigm case is someone like Karen Quinlan, who has reached a mature age that allows those close to her to know her likely wishes, a case like that of Saikewicz requires that others stand in his place and reason to what his judgment would have been, based on our own best judgment of his best interest. Of course, we can never know what his actual preferences would have been, so a "substituted judgment" standard is likely to be inherently more uncertain and correspondingly subject to greater criticism. Invoking an ideal of justice as fairness, critics of the court's decision might reasonably argue that his intellectual disability should not have created a presumption that the burdens of chemotherapy would be greater for him than for others or the extension of his life for a few more months any less valuable.

In challenging situations like those presented by end-of-life care, our ethical understanding doesn't flow purely from principles (simple deduction) or detailed case studies (simple intuition). Ethical casuistry at its best moves from presumptive principles and paradigms to complex real cases and back again. Its basic premise—that "virtue is incomplete without the skill of practical deliberation"—reflects how many bioethicists reason through hard cases, even if they wouldn't say they are practicing casuistry, any more than they would say they are speaking prose. To advance publicly defensible policies, the ethical debates over physician-assisted death cry out for us to consider both well-established principles and paradigm cases.

Two other methods in bioethics call attention to features of Joseph Saikewicz's predicament that may not be fully captured by appeal to principles or through a casuistic analysis. Feminist bioethics is critical of rigid principles that don't adequately attend to aspects of gender, power, and class in the way that health care is delivered. This view calls upon us to consider whether the decisions we propose to make for Saikewicz are truly in his interest, taking full account of his necessary dependency on others. And it also calls upon us to understand whether or how those interests would be different for patients capable of self-determination.

The care perspective in bioethics similarly emphasizes the utter vulnerability of someone in his position, and the responsibilities we all have to care for others (and others have to care for us). No man or woman is an island, but emphasizing individual rights above social responsibilities or duties to others can be misleading in making it seem that way. In elaborating these details of the Saikeweicz case, we have introduced aspects of his story that call attention to the person in his particular, radically dependent situation rather than only to ethical principles as applied to any abstract individual.

FROM "DEBBIE" TO "DR. DEATH"ʼ

In 1988 the *Journal of the American Medical Association* published an unsigned item entitled "It's Over, Debbie," purporting to describe a dying patient in a hospital. Allegedly written by an exhausted young doctor, the narrative tells us that twenty-year-old Debbie is terminally ill from ovarian cancer and, having failed chemotherapy, is experiencing severe vomiting. Called to the bedside from another part of the hospital in the middle of the night, the doctor notes the patient's labored breathing. Another, older woman holds Debbie's hand. Debbie appears to be in very poor condition with anorexia and insomnia, and her only words to the doctor were "Let's get this over with." Retreating to the nurse's station, the writer recalls thinking, "I could not give her health, but I could give her rest." Injecting morphine sulfate into a syringe, "enough, I thought, to do the job," the doctor reentered the room and told Debbie that this "would let her rest and . . . say good-bye." As her breathing became normal she appeared to rest, the older woman stroking her hair. "With clocklike certainty, within four minutes the breathing rate slowed even more, then became irregular, then ceased. The dark-haired woman stood erect and seemed relieved." The piece concluded, "It's over, Debbie."

"It's Over, Debbie" provoked vigorous protests at several levels.

First, physician ethicists objected to the impression that it might give that death-dealing drugs are administered so casually in hospitals, without considering the informed consent of patients, while quite the reverse is the case. Second, many observed that the piece was an obvious hoax, not only because of some very odd references (an "alcohol drip"), but also the remarkable vagueness about who the people were in the room and what they really wanted. Third, there were objections about the ethics of journalism in the editor's very decision to publish such a flawed and misleading screed. All agreed that this was a worst-case scenario—a negative paradigm—for aid-in-dying.

The controversy over "Debbie" was all the more striking because it came at nearly the same time that a Michigan pathologist named Jack Kevorkian, whose name would become a lightning rod in the 1990s, started advertising his "death counseling" services in Detroit newspapers. In 1990, two years after the "Debbie" publication, he helped a fifty-four-year-old woman named Janet Adkins die by hooking her up to a "Thanatron," or death machine, in the back of his Volkswagen bus. Adkins had been diagnosed with Alzheimer's disease. Like nearly all of Kevorkian's 130 clients, or victims, from 1990 to 1998, Adkins herself set in motion the chemical system of sodium thiopental and potassium chloride. Some people who sought Kevorkian's aid were not terminally ill and did not report pain, and others had only met him a day before he provided the means of their death.

Kevorkian was a complicated, and troubling, character. Some bioethicists were familiar with him long before he burst on the scene for his death counseling. For years he had advocated that death row prisoners be allowed to choose to subject themselves to medical experimentation over execution. The notion was macabre and incompatible with the widely honored and established ethical norms. But Kevorkian, eager for the spotlight, was nothing if not persistent. Known to many as "Dr. Death," Kevorkian became a kind of culture hero to some, while a death-peddling, law-defying villain to others. Public efforts to promote laws allowing physician aid-in-dying were not new. An organization called the Hemlock Society was succeeded by Compassion & Choices, but Kevorkian's approach was radical, and by conventional standards clearly unethical, going far beyond anything advocated by established organizations. Aiding "suffering or doomed persons [to] kill themselves" was, in his own words, "merely the first step":

> What I find most satisfying is the prospect of making possible the performance of invaluable experiments or other beneficial medical acts under conditions that this first unpleasant step can help establish.

Whether Kevorkian was aware of it or not, his fanatical character and uncompromising sense of mission played well into media fascination with what he considered his conscientious objection. Matters came to a head in 1998, when Kevorkian allowed the CBS news program *60 Minutes* to broadcast a tape of his injecting Thomas Youk, a fifty-two-year-old man with Lou Gehrig's disease. Kevorkian was found guilty of second-degree murder and sentenced to prison. After eight years he was paroled for good behavior and died in 2011. By then Kevorkian had undeniably become a culture hero to some Americans, however unlikely, and the subject of a popular and award-winning biopic starring Al Pacino. But his careless approach—and the fact that his "patients" were used as part of what was in effect a macabre performance of death—undermined his message of compassion.

THE CASE OF DIANE

For anyone who appreciates the gravity of ending a human life, the Debbie essay represents one extreme of unethical physician-assisted death, if indeed the incident took place at all. For Kevorkian's many critics, his "treatment" was only marginally superior to simply walking into an unfamiliar patient's room, seeing that she is suffering or terminally ill, and giving her a lethal injection. After Debbie and during the rise of awareness about Kevorkian's campaign, many Americans wondered whether an ethically plausible alternative existed to these cases, one that was a paradigm example of physician-assisted death at the other, positive side of the moral spectrum. To many, that example was provided by Timothy Quill, a physician from Rochester, New York, whose story was brought to light in the pages of another important medical publication, the *New England Journal of Medicine*, in 1991.

For some years, Quill had cared for a forty-five-year-old patient he called "Diane." Knowing that she had been through a previous bout of cancer and aware of her difficult childhood in an alcoholic household and her struggles with her own alcoholism and depression, he felt he knew her as a strong, determined person. Quill also had extensive experience with cancer patients as a former hospice program director and primary care physician, so when Diane was diagnosed with myelomonocytic leukemia, he was prepared to counsel her as an informed doctor. Diane's treatment would have involved chemotherapy, bone marrow transplants, whole-body irradiation, and lengthy hospitalization, with a 25 percent survival rate. According to Quill, she had long discussions with her husband and son about her decision not to pursue treatment, preferring to live whatever time remained with them.

At first Quill, who supported patients' rights to die with dignity, arranged for home hospice care. Medical treatment would be limited to measures that would keep Diane comfortable. But Diane decided that she preferred to control the timing of her death. After assuring himself that this was not an act of desperation or a manifestation of her previous depression and that Diane had the capacity to make her own decision, Quill provided her with a prescription for barbiturates for insomnia with the understanding that an overdose would result in her death. When the time came, Diane insisted that no one else be present when she took the medication so that no one else would be legally implicated. As Quill wrote later, the fact that Diane died alone was his one source of regret.

Like Kevorkian, Quill also faced legal issues. He had, after all, reported that he had prescribed medication to a patient with the full knowledge that she might well use it to take her life. And he had done so in a most public manner, in the pages of an elite medical journal. Unlike Kevorkian, the results of Quill's intervention were not nearly as dire. After several hours of testimony, a few months after the journal article appeared, a grand jury in Rochester chose not to criminally indict him. Those who adamantly opposed physician involvement in hastening a patient's death were certainly not convinced that this legal outcome settled the ethical issue.

The case also left many otherwise sympathetic bioethicists uneasy, including some of those who were inclined to see Quill's handling of the Diane case as far more ethically justifiable than the early actions of Kevorkian and those reported in the short essay about "Debbie." They asked: By giving implicit support of Diane's right to end her life, was Quill helping to create an atmosphere in which physician-assisted death would become more common but without the mitigating elements of the case of Diane? Many of those otherwise sympathetic to Diane's plight worried about such a "slippery slope," including both the implications for those who were not truly capable of making the decision to end their own lives and the doctors who, they feared, would be far too cooperative with them.

SLIPPERY SLOPES

Slippery slope arguments are among the most common in discussions about public policy, but it's important to understand their ethical limitations. Intended to oppose the introduction of a new policy, the assertion that "X might lead to Y" typically conceals more than it brings to light. Assuming that Y is ethically unacceptable, the assertion doesn't require agreement that X is also unacceptable. "Life," as columnist George Will writes, "is inevitably lived on multiple slippery slopes":

> Taxation could become confiscation, police could become instruments of oppression, public education could become indoctrination, etc. Everywhere and always, civilization depends on the drawing of intelligent distinctions.

Will is an especially compelling critic of slippery slope arguments on this subject because he is also a staunch defender of the sanctity of life. Yet he rejects slippery slope arguments against "death with dignity" laws that respect patient autonomy and are regulated to avoid abuse. The Oregon law does not mistake treating patient liberty or autonomy for license. Instead, it balances respect for patient autonomy with requirements to help ensure beneficence and protect against maleficence. The opposing slippery slope arguments suggest that *any* law authorizing physician-assisted death, no matter how carefully crafted, will unacceptably exacerbate an absolutely indefensible culture of casual death.

Slippery slope arguments tend to bypass the consideration of a policy on its own merits. However valuable it is to allow competent adults like Maynard to engage "in affirming at the end the distinctive human dignity of autonomous choice," the slippery slope argument suggests that what predictably follows will be obviously worse. The legalization of physician-assisted death is presumed to lead downstream to something so bad—such as involuntary euthanasia—that it obviates the need to weigh the uncertain future bad against the certain present good. These predictions are highly uncertain, yet they are presented in a way that elides the core moral question: Under what circumstances, if any, is it ethical for a physician to prescribe a life-terminating medication to a terminally ill patient?

Since slippery slope arguments predict that even the most carefully crafted laws will lead to something so bad that it's worth overriding a patient's autonomy, we need to ask: How well-founded is the prediction of the bad consequently to come? In the decades since the earliest cases we've been discussing, the passage of state laws permitting physician-assisted death has turned in no small part on successfully avoiding multiple slippery slopes. This becomes clear when we look back at the way that physician aid-in-dying laws have developed in the United States. (The experience of some other countries is more mixed, as we will see.)

A critical consideration for state legal systems has been how to permit a narrow range of factors that can justify physician-assisted death while drawing clear boundaries to avoid abuse. Typically, state laws require a multistep certification process before approving a patient request, confirmed by witnesses (one of whom has no conflict of interest); a second physician must confirm the diagnosis and prognosis; the patient must make oral and written requests; and the patient must be offered hospice.

When Oregon voters became the first to approve a "death with dignity" act in 1994, another key element was a provision respecting the right of any health care provider with a conscientious objection not to participate in the practice. It's an intriguing—and revealing—fact that more American doctors say that they want access to physician-assisted death for themselves than would be willing to provide such assistance to a patient (well-informed, like themselves). Thinking of themselves as patients, these doctors would want the option of a physician-assisted "death with dignity." But in their role as doctors, they oppose legalizing the practice even if they are exempted from professionally participating in it. While doctors who oppose the practice often trace their opposition back to the Hippocratic precept "first, do no harm," the precept can be reasonably interpreted as an injunction not to harm terminally ill patients by overriding their well-informed ethical sensibility of how to end their lives with dignity. The fact that this sensibility is shared by many doctors is at least an implicit concession of the reasonableness of the (nonphysician) patients who seek it.

Death with dignity laws take account of dissenting doctors and admirably respect their conscience, analogous to how doctors can and (we think) should respect the conscience of informed patients (including some doctors themselves) to seek physician-assisted death from a doctor who approves of the practice. All U.S. states that have passed laws permitting physician-assisted death include this exception for dissenting doctors along with strict guardrails, thereby respecting both the autonomy of competent adult patients who are terminally ill and the right of physicians not to participate if they morally object to the practice.

By making the conditions of legalization stringent and specific, defenders of physician-assisted death have managed to develop a strongly favorable consensus in states that have adopted these laws. Efforts to overturn or cripple them through both proposed federal and state legislation and legal challenges, including one that made it up to the U.S. Supreme Court, have failed.

KEEPING WATCH

While the guardrails erected in the American context to prevent slippage from physician-assisted death so far have proven quite secure, the track records of some other countries are more questionable. Although we generally support physician aid-in-dying laws under the kinds of conditions we've described, we are also committed to closely observing any evidence of abuse, whether in the United States or abroad. As compared to the statutes in the U.S. jurisdictions, some of the arrangements that have been approved in some European countries strike many as riper for abuse and help to confirm some of the worst fears of those who want doctors to have nothing to do with hastening the end of life at all.

Among the controversial examples is the Netherlands, which allows not only physician assistance but also active euthanasia to be requested by patients starting at age twelve (though up to sixteen only with parental consent). There are no age requirements in Belgium so long as the patient is found by a psychiatrist or psychologist to have the capacity for understanding and judgment (*capacite de discernment*), is suffering unbearable physical pain, and all this is certified in writing. A particular flash point in any form of assisted death is the question of whether a chronically depressed person has the ability to make that decision if all therapies have failed. In Belgium, only adults may qualify for euthanasia based on mental suffering. A critical question—if one accepts the general proposition that supports physician-assisted death—is whether the patient's psychological condition is interfering with their ability to make a decision that truly reflects their values and preferences. The answer surely requires a case-by-case assessment, guided by principled respect for each person's values and preferences as best they can be discerned. As ethical casuistry and an ethics of care would suggest, there's no formulaic deduction that can reliably be applied to decide every case.

It is also important not to overgeneralize about the situation in various countries. Switzerland, for example, has permitted doctors to prescribe lethal drugs for medical illness since 1942, whether or not the patient is a Swiss citizen. In spite of that long tradition, Switzerland is not thought of as a hotbed of suicide tourism. The Netherlands has become more well-known not only because of its highly public discussion of physician-assisted death and its policy of official tolerance if certain conditions are fulfilled (unbearable suffering with no prospect of improvement is one of them) but most likely because of its policy on infant euthanasia. The Groningen Protocol is named for the medical center whose director led the policy's development in the early 2000s. Following meetings of a group at Groningen and various consultations, the protocol permits infants to be actively killed if, besides hopeless and unbearable suffering that has been medically confirmed, the parents give consent and the procedure is done with care, along with other criteria. Perhaps no single policy on physician aid-in-dying has provoked more controversy than the Groningen Protocol. Opponents, including the Roman Catholic Church, argue that the protocol is little more than a medicalized excuse for murdering socially burdensome babies. Though doctors who follow its provisions are not guaranteed that they won't be prosecuted, the Dutch pediatric association has endorsed it and a number of cases have been reported.

We are still in search of evidence of serious slippage. So far, there seems to be strong cultural resistance to Groningen even in places that have legalized some form of medically assisted death, usually short of active euthanasia, for patients who are legal adults. That list of states and countries has grown in Western Europe and North America, with Canada recently added and Colombia in South America. Most data in the United States come from Oregon and Washington, where most requests are associated with cancer, and patients tend to be older, white, well educated, and well insured. Pain avoidance is typically not the major factor, according to the information that's available; loss of dignity and quality of life are.

Have the rules been abused? The best available evidence suggests that not many cases in the United States go beyond the guidelines we've described. That could be because abuses aren't being reported and can't be identified in other ways. Were rule breaking widespread, however, it would be hard to conceal. In any case, evidence-based conclusions about rule breaking would require careful comparisons of the incidence of abuse between places that have legalized physician-assisted death and those that don't. After all, the basic hypothesis of any such investigation is that it is rash to simply assume that people will abide by the law. The experience of Oregon, at a minimum, suggests that death with dignity laws can respect not only the dignity and autonomy of patients but also the beneficence and nonmaleficence of physicians. However, critics and defenders alike have worried that if physician-assisted death becomes a routine practice, members of marginalized and vulnerable groups will be pressured to end their lives, especially if their families are in financial distress or there are opportunities for compensated organ donation. That nightmare scenario should be guarded against with good guidelines and rigorous reporting.

COMPETING CONCEPTS OF DIGNITY

Although surveys show that large majorities approve of physician-assisted death, many conscientious people—including many doctors—directly oppose it as a matter of principle. They will not be satisfied with the most stringent conditions on its practice. Their disagreement is ethically deep, resting upon a competing interpretation of dignity. Bioethicist Daniel Sulmasy calls it "intrinsic dignity" and in practice he conceives it as trumping (and ethically refuting) Maynard's own sense of what it means to end her own life with dignity. As Sulmasy puts the case against physician-assisted death: "Intending that somebody be turned into a nobody violates the fundamental basis of our interpersonal ethics, our intrinsic dignity." Sulmasy also interprets autonomy in a way that rejects the idea that we should respect the freedom of a competent adult to end her life: "saying that respect for liberty justifies the obliteration of liberty actually undermines the value that we place on human freedom."

Some principled opponents of physician-assisted death, like Sulmasy, strongly support life-terminating palliative care as long as it is *intended* to relieve the pain of terminally ill patients even when the predictable outcome of the prescribed (or even physician-administered) medication is the patient's death. What's morally prohibited, they argue, is not *ending* a person's freedom forever, but rather their *intending to end* it. They draw upon a doctrine of "double effect," whose lineage dates back to Thomas Aquinas's *Summa Theologica*.

According to double effect, one can justify *the first intended effect* of alleviating unbearable pain of a terminally ill person through palliative care even if *the second unintended effect* is death, provided that the positive value of the intended pain relief outweighs the negative value of the unintended shortening of life. To understand what's distinctive about double effect, we need to go beyond the fact that, like other defenses of life-terminating palliative care with a patient's informed consent, it, too, requires that on balance there be positive pain-relieving benefits to shortening a patient's life. Double effect holds that there can be no death with dignity *if the intended action— even if it is undertaken by a fully competent patient without any medical assistance—is to cause death in order to relieve unbearable end-of-life suffering.* Why? Because on this conception, the dignity of human life is violated by an intent to end one's life, to make oneself a "nobody" rather than a "somebody." Defenders of carefully constrained death with dignity laws, by contrast, think that human dignity depends at least in part on the considered judgment of individuals who face end-of-life decisions. They (and we) think that respecting a terminally ill patient's final autonomous wish—to die with dignity—is justifiable under some conditions.

This is about as basic a conflict of perspectives as we get in ethics, and it is important to recognize, as some defenses of death with dignity seem to deny, that no position is neutral in this debate. Those who place a high value on autonomy, for example, will defend Brittany Maynard's position: society should give others who may find themselves "walking in her shoes" the same choices that she had. But there's nothing ethically neutral about respect for individual autonomy. We deeply respect those doctors like Sulmasy who find physician-assisted death (which they call assisted suicide) morally impermissible, and we would want democratically authorized legislation to respect everyone's right not to participate. But we argue that it can be ethical, and it should be legal, for competent adults who find themselves "walking a mile" in Maynard's shoes to use their last free act to die with dignity, as they reasonably interpret it. This concept of human dignity can consistently affirm the idea that intentionally acting to end one's life is not always wrong. Every human life, after all, has a last act.

The claim to death with dignity is often paired in academic writings with an argument for individual autonomy. Compared to dignity, autonomy is a more precisely developed concept in modern philosophy, but in a variety of ways dignity plays a distinctively important role in public debates about the ethics of end-of-life care. Many proponents appeal to dignity as one justification for limiting aid-in-dying to health care professionals, both because a medical framework lends legitimacy to the act—an outcome that is deeply worrisome to opponents—and because when professionally prescribed, drugs are more likely to be used correctly, making it less likely that a patient will end up in even worse condition.

What about the argument that death with dignity laws are unnecessary because terminal sedation (also called "medical death") can relieve a patient of her suffering? Double effect can support terminal sedation as long as its intention is to relieve suffering, not to kill the patient. (Medical death is so-called because it will predictably—but not intentionally—kill the patient, hence the "double effect.") Defenders of physician-assisted death respond that many competent people are appalled by the idea of being forced to end their lives slowly in a totally dependent, unconscious condition when there exists a more humane and dignified alternative. Again, the best available data from the United States show that most patients seeking physician-assisted death say they are motivated by the loss of dignity, autonomy, and their inability to enjoy life, and not primarily by pain avoidance.

Since the idea of dignity admits strongly competing concepts—and is significantly more ambiguous than respect for persons—why continue to invoke it in debating life-and-death issues? The bioethicist Ruth Macklin has argued that dignity is a poorly defined slogan, when it is defined at all, and adds nothing to the bioethics principle of respect for persons or autonomy. Her argument triggered an important debate, which helps illuminate competing conceptions of dignity. Even if respect for persons and autonomy best captures its moral meaning, dignity is still a valuable concept in our world. A broad idea (not unlike respect for persons), dignity has an important role to play, especially in public deliberations where it's almost always a mistake to let the perfect be the enemy of the good. For a start, dignity reminds us that the status of being human has a special place in our history, our existential condition, and our ethical life. Its usage can be traced at least as far back as Socrates and religious traditions that conceive of human beings as created equal and capable of thinking for themselves and of acting to avoid being agents of injustice.

A practical reason not to let dignity go by the wayside in a bioethical argument is that international human rights documents appeal to respect for human dignity as a core value. In addition, as we have seen, dignity plays a significant public role in guiding attempts to adapt to the proliferation of medical technologies that can extend life but cannot restore the gravely ill to a life they deem worth living. Rather than cede "dignity" as a term to those who devalue individual autonomy, we respect its substantial role in creating an overlapping consensus on important public policies such as physician-assisted death.

COMING TO TERMS

How do we want to die? Since the birth of modern bioethics in the developed world, the line of cases from letting die to physician aid-in-dying to active euthanasia has resulted in a broad consensus in favor of less aggressive treatment of terminally ill patients, some acceptance of physician assistance (as in the cases of Brittany Maynard and Diane), and significant resistance to active euthanasia (especially in the Debbie case and Jack Kevorkian's lethal injection of Thomas Youk). To us, this trend represents our collective attempt to come to terms with the changing roles of doctors and patients coupled with the increasing ability of modern medical technologies to extend human life but sometimes in a state that some people reasonably decide is not worth living. Yet this trend of ceding terminally ill patients the legal ability to obtain a physician-assisted death is not universal. Most southern hemisphere societies have not publicly tackled this issue. Central and Eastern Europe have been described as places where support for medically assisted death is decreasing.

If everybody recognizes the certainty of dying, we certainly don't agree on how best to die, even under similar circumstances. Amid our disagreement over physician-assisted death, we can understand competing conceptions of human dignity along with differing approaches to end-of-life care and their policy implications. This understanding not only helps us respect our opponents on this issue while we continue our deep disagreement, it also offers a productive path to cultivating some vitally important common ground.

In coming to terms with the debate over physician-assisted death, we touched upon the common ground that opponents can productively cultivate. Although we disagree with Sulmasy about physician-assisted death/suicide (even over what to call it), we join forces in advocating for access to affordable hospice and palliative care. Affordability for all patients, so often neglected in the practice of American medicine, is a key issue. So much of modern medicine focuses on extending life, too often to the neglect of dealing with death as "an intrinsic element of our humanity." For death to be experienced with dignity, everyone should be informed about their most caring and comforting options, and they should be able to afford those options. Millions more lives stand to be improved by better educating health care professionals and everyone who wants to know about end-of-life care options that importantly include hospice and palliative care. This is a crucial first step, and just as crucially it needs to be followed by meeting the ensuing public demand for affordable and effective hospice care and other high-quality palliative treatment. A large proportion of Americans may want and need hospice at the end of their lives; its prospects for success in relieving physical, mental, and spiritual suffering are high; its costs are moderate to low; and it serves the common good of compassionately caring for one another.

The rapid development of the hospice care movement in the United States, which only began in the 1960s, offers hope for cultivating this common ground. Hospice came into demand in an environment in which new medical technologies proliferated with the power to extend lives without regard to quality of life. It has rapidly expanded as a worldwide movement. Where hospice is known to be accessible and affordable, it has become widely accepted and chosen by ever-increasing numbers of terminally ill patients. Yet for all this progress, surveys show that most Americans—including about a third of the elderly and chronically ill—have never discussed life-and-death decisions with a health care provider. A minority of providers have had training in how to conduct such discussions. Cultivating this common ground depends on significantly expanding the scope of health care education and communication.

In the cauldron of a highly polarized democratic politics, one of the greatest challenges to cultivating common ground is finding pathways that mitigate the potential damage done by ruthless efforts to spread falsehoods that render one's political adversaries into one's mortal enemies. A prime example of this damage occurred when the 2009 bill that would become the Affordable Care Act (aka Obamacare) proposed covering voluntary discussions between patients and doctors about end-of-life care options. The baseless claim by former Alaska governor and vice presidential candidate Sarah Palin that the federal government was trying to create "death panels" that would decide whether to "pull the plug on Grandma," as a senator put it, quickly gained traction through the news and social media. Immediate damage was done to a health care bill without bipartisan support that was teetering on the brink of political defeat; the provision was pulled from the bill. But proponents of the provision did not give up on what could be common ground. Six years later, after relentlessly countering the falsehoods and finding broad public support for the provision, the Centers for Medicare and Medicaid Services in the Obama administration passed a rule that requires Medicare to pay for voluntary patient-doctor discussions of end-of-life care. In being explicit that end-of-life planning occurs only "at the discretion of the beneficiary," the rule makes absolutely clear its proponents' intention both to counter the falsehoods and to cultivate this common ground.

Finding a way forward for the American government to fund voluntary end-of-life discussions between patients and doctors is not cause to declare either ethical or political victory in Americans' coming to terms with how we want to die. But it is cause for believing that with greater willingness to search openly and honestly for such ground, we can find more ways forward. We must begin—but not end—by expanding thoughtful, evidence-based public debate and deliberation about the hardest subject known to human beings: how to come to ethical terms—collectively as well as individually—with our own mortality.

Five

THE HIGH PRICE
OF UNFAIR
HEALTH CARE

Before Medicare and Medicaid were passed in 1965, health spending for the poorest 20 percent of Americans was less than for all other groups, despite the fact that they are generally also in worse health than those with higher incomes. According to a group of health economists, by 1977 spending increased for the poorest including millions of children, an indicator that they were finally getting more of the health care they needed. However, by 2004 that favorable trend reversed. The unfavorable trend has persisted, with health care spending for the highest income 20 percent rising by 20 percent. Moreover, U.S. life expectancy declined in 2015 for the first time in 20 years. Economists Anne Case and Angus Deaton had warned for years that rates of death and illness among middle-aged whites were increasing.

This health care picture is consistent with rapidly growing income inequality in the United States since the 1970s. In every succeeding decade, the middle class shrank while the wealth gap between middle- and upper-income groups widened dramatically, with black Americans and the elderly still most likely to be low income. The decade of the Great Recession hit lower-income groups the hardest. By 2015, for the first time on record, more American adults were in the lowest and highest income groups combined; the middle class was no longer a majority in America. This trend, President Barack

Obama argued in his last State of the Union address, threatens the social fabric of the country. Evidence for that argument ranges from the opioid epidemic that has especially impacted lower-income white Americans to the election of Donald Trump in 2016, whose campaign rhetoric conveyed that the American dream had been stolen by immigrants, foreign countries (including U.S. allies), and drowned in the swamp of the political establishment, threatening Americans' lives and livelihoods; only he could fix it.

While promising to "drain the swamp," some political leaders argue that it's time to cut back on the "safety net" of health care and welfare programs that protect the most vulnerable. This perverse and cruel policy not only ignores the facts but, we argue, also exacerbates the unfairness of a system that expects people to work but deprives them of the health care they may need to get or hold a job and to pursue just about every other opportunity in life. Cutting back on health insurance is also a disconcerting retreat from the era when Americans, once confronted with the limits of their country's resources, found better ways to arrange a health care financing system that was more equitable even if still less than ideal.

LIBERALS, LIBERTARIANS, AND UTILITARIANS

In threatening times we need to shine a spotlight on values that inform popular debates in the United States about government's role in advancing health care. A large family of liberal perspectives supports government subsidies of health care for all those who need it but cannot otherwise afford it. Why? Multiple answers converge on broadly similar policy prescriptions. The Rawlsian perspective developed by Norman Daniels views affordable health care as essential to fair equality of opportunity. Amartya Sen's "capabilities" perspective sees health care as an essential enabler. It gives people the capacity to do all the other basic and important things in their lives. Importantly, a right to health care is also compatible with respecting the fundamental individual freedoms of speech, religion, citizenship, and so on. Like education, health care is necessary for everyone to enjoy everything else that's important in life.

By liberal lights, health care is a basic human right and the failure of an affluent society to fund universal access to affordable health care is a blatant injustice, and an avoidable one. Affordable health care in the United States remains inaccessible to millions—in contrast to Canada, the United Kingdom, France, Germany, Japan, Australia, South Korea, and almost every other industrialized country and many less affluent ones as well! Millions of America's poorer residents are either uninsured or underinsured.

The absence of U.S. government funding for universal health care draws support from the radically libertarian perspective of Robert Nozick, which seems to resonate with significant parts of the American public especially when it comes to redistributive taxation. Nozick opposed governmental redistribution for the sake of health care because (in his words) "taxation of earnings from labor is on a par with forced labor." By these libertarian lights, taxation to pay for some people's health care unjustly usurps other people's hard-earned money. This is a radical position even in a country whose revolution was made in the name of freedom from taxation *without representation*. Nozick's position, which translates into the contemporary Tea Party's adamant opposition to government funding of health care, calls for freedom from taxation *even with representation*.

The more moderate and famous libertarian, F. A. Hayek, in his best-selling *The Road to Serfdom*, makes significantly greater exceptions to freedom from taxation, strongly advocating for government's role in ensuring the health, education, and safety of all. Although more often celebrated for opposing overweening governments that stifle individual freedom, Hayek vehemently rejected what he called a "dogmatic laissez faire attitude." He staunchly supported social insurance to protect people from the scourge of illness:

Where, as in the case of sickness and accident, neither the desire to avoid such calamities nor the efforts to overcome their consequences are as a rule weakened by the provision of assistance, where in short, we deal with genuinely insurable risks, the case for the state's helping to organize a comprehensive system of social insurance is very strong.

Utilitarians invoke the philosophy that originated with Jeremy Bentham when they defend universal health insurance as a policy that maximizes social welfare: gross benefits minus costs to society and individuals. By first principle, utilitarianism is cost-conscious— no wonder that economists and economically-minded Americans find it such an appealing perspective. It calls on governments to choose those health care programs that yield the greatest positive social return. Utilitarianism comes with its share of moral controversy: attempts to maximize social welfare can be used in ways that yield socially unacceptable results, as we'll see in the case of the Seattle "life-and-death committee." But combining a careful cost-benefit calculation with considerations of fairness and basic human rights provides a way of making the most out of scarcity.

THE SHOCK OF THE SCARCE

In the 1950s few Americans doubted their country's ability to make good stuff, and plenty of it, forever. The country's productivity during World War II was remarkable. At the outbreak of the war, factories that made cars and trucks were seemingly overnight turned into factories that made tanks and landing craft. A vast industry of naval vessels sprang up in rapidly expanded ports. Many armaments were manufactured and sent to the Russian front, on the other side of the world, with plenty remaining for Americans fighting in Europe and the Pacific. The "arsenal of democracy" was at full strength.

On the medical side, the White House created a special office to evaluate and fund innovations that could support the war effort, from new drugs for diseases like malaria to improvements in procedures like blood transfusion. If there were shortages in "miracle drugs" like penicillin, at least one could be assured that those shortages were temporary. The unspoken assumption—needed health care would somehow be made universally affordable and accessible—is as unwarranted now as it was then. One major change is that the question "Who gets access to what lifesaving and life-extending medicines and health care?" in our childhoods largely was posed (if at all) sotto voce, behind closed doors, invisible then to the vast majority of Americans.

Before the age of the internet and social media, fewer and slower means of communication meant less public awareness of two sides of the scarcity equation: the magnitudes of both the deprivations due to scarcity and the costs of scaling up to overcome it. An odd by-product of the growth of our knowledge about illness is an appreciation of the obstacles to producing a technical solution, especially in large numbers. Sometimes a desired resource is scarce not because it's actually rare, like precious metals, but because it's just expensive and difficult to make a lot of it. This is the difference between natural and artificial scarcity. When a costly lifesaving cure for a disease is first discovered, the path to producing enough to treat everybody afflicted by the illness is likely blocked by some natural scarcities—human organs for transplant being the classic example—but most blockages consist of decisions or neglect about devoting the financial and human resources needed to treat all potential beneficiaries.

Artificial scarcity in any realm that puts many lives at risk has the potential to produce a sense of public crisis once it's publicized, like the crisis of the delay of food distribution to the Hurricane Katrina flood victims in 2005. Shining a public spotlight on victims of artificial scarcity brings public compassion to the fore and elicits a sense of moral outrage to the extent that the scarcity is connected to a clearly avoidable injustice. Hurricanes epitomize the devastating fury of nature, but there was nothing either natural or necessary about the devastating delays in delivering food, water, shelter, and health care to hurricane victims. When public light shines on artificial scarcity in the realm of lifesaving health care goods and services, a sense of crisis is often not far behind. Averting such crises before they happen calls for the cultivation and exercise of civic virtues whose scarce supply also is artificial. A sense of the common good can inform deliberations about hard choices, as in the production and distribution of lifesaving resources.

The iconic black bags that we associated with the kindly doctors of our childhood were not the bottomless baskets of bread and fish of the Sermon on the Mount. And if one actually did an analysis, the doctors with those black bags visited disproportionately more white than black children, but that kind of de facto inequality was rarely observed. Most of the victims of artificial health care scarcity, then as now, have had no public spotlight shone on them. We as humans are both shortsighted (overvaluing the present) and nearsighted (identifying with those more akin to oneself). We fail to focus on the diverse millions who lack adequate health care coverage. Some may not be in vividly dire straits but one day they will be, having been deprived of adequate health care. The United States has made progress, in fits and starts, over decades in affording needed health care to a larger proportion of Americans. But significant artificial scarcity of health care resources continues, not only in the United States but worldwide, and therefore so does the urgency that we all attend to who gets access to what health care.

THEY DECIDE WHO LIVES

Before the Salk vaccine was developed, the iron lung aided children with polio whose disease had progressed to a dangerous stage—a lifesaving but scary object (as we discussed in chapter 3). And they were the lucky ones. At the time, many Americans may not have appreciated that iron lungs were rationed; few publicly questioned how they were rationed. The next lifesaving device—a precious few artificial kidney machines—got the country's attention. For the whole of human history, people whose kidneys stopped working died of the excess salt, water, and waste products unleashed on their bodies. Finally, during World War II, a Dutch physician started work on an artificial kidney for short-term use. Nearly twenty years later, in 1960, Belding Scribner, an American doctor at the University of Washington, developed a machine for long-term dialysis. Patients who would otherwise have died of end-stage renal disease came to Seattle's Swedish Hospital twice a week and spent as much as sixteen hours having their blood cleansed by circulating it through the machine in Teflon tubes. As long as they stuck to a restricted diet, they could live normal lives.

But not all patients. From the beginning, it was obvious that the demand for time on dialysis could easily overwhelm the hospital, and indeed any place with significant numbers of patients. Treating one patient for a year cost over $120,000 in today's dollars. At that time, there were perhaps two thousand qualified patients in the United States. How to decide who among them should receive the treatment? The hospital appointed a committee, assigning its members the vital but unenviable task of deciding. An anonymous committee of local citizens, seven volunteers who served without pay, was charged with deciding who would get access to the machine: a lawyer, a minister, a banker, a housewife, a state government official, a labor leader, and a surgeon. The committee acted as a kind of ethical buffer between the "medical men" and the desperate patients. Only a few out of all those who applied for renal dialysis could be accepted, a limit justified by the hospital's leadership because the dialysis program was a kind of experimental trial. The committee was given only two other guidelines: patients over forty-five were bad medical risks and children should be excluded, as they would have a hard time tolerating the treatment.

In 1962 millions of Americans read the remarkable story of this "life-and-death committee" in an article in *Life* magazine by the renowned journalist Shana Alexander. It was the prosperous beginning of what the press dubbed the "soaring '60s." How their society should deal with medical scarcity, or scarcity of any kind, wasn't something most post-WWII Americans had been encouraged let alone taught to think much about, though millions of their fellow citizens lived in grinding poverty. In spite of the lack of guidelines and the seemingly arbitrary nature of the decisions—was a younger woman with six children to be favored over an older woman with three?—Alexander found that the committee acted with a high degree of consensus. They considered just drawing straws, but they ruled that out, thinking it their responsibility to find a nonrandom basis for selection. The factors they explicitly considered included the patient's marital status, number of dependents, net worth, occupation, education, church attendance, and potential to resume work. These factors seemed to be surrogates for determining—on roughly utilitarian grounds—whose life was most "worth" saving and whose death the least "costly"—all things considered—to society. Once brought to public light, the very idea of a health care jury assessing each person's relative worth in comparison to others, for the sake of making a life-and-death decision, was highly controversial.

While no one doubted the committee's good intentions or public-regarding motives, their decisions had an unsettling morally arbitrary dimension—utilitarian considerations of maximizing social welfare notwithstanding. One of the strongest criticisms was not that they were using the *wrong* person-specific considerations of worthiness, or aggregate social welfare, but that they were using *any* such considerations except potential receptivity to the medical treatment itself. As Alexander ruefully observed, "on the basis of the past year's record, a candidate who plans to come before this committee would seem well-advised to father a great many children, then to throw away all his money, and finally to fall ill in a season when there will be a minimum of competition from other men dying of the same disease."

The article and the facts surrounding the Seattle "life-and-death committee" are credited with sparking widespread national attention and interest in bioethics. The case study was a favorite of early bioethics courses. It represents, in a simplified and purified form, similar underlying issues to the ones we still face in deciding who should get access to scarce health care goods and services, and at what price. Decades later we each taught it in different courses to diverse students. It always ignited our students' interest in understanding the practical implications of competing ethical perspectives. It also made manifest that the ethical perspectives of decision makers have life-and-death consequences, and for many people. One of the committee member's comments to Alexander could easily be expressed today: "We send billions of dollars overseas to people we know nothing about, many of whom despise us. If Congress or somebody wanted to provide the money, we could take care of all our kidney people. But where do we stop? . . . I frankly don't know." Decisions today about how much government should do to provide access to health care have become even more challenging as medicine's lifesaving capacity and health care costs have exponentially increased.

The shortage of dialysis machines for every qualified end-stage kidney disease patient was an issue until October 1972 when President Richard Nixon signed an omnibus Social Security bill into law that included a little-debated provision extending Medicare coverage to all victims of end-stage renal disease, a bill for which the disgraced Nixon is rarely given credit. The Senate (which prided itself on being the greatest deliberative body in the world) debated the amendment for thirty minutes. Only one senator spoke against it, and fifty-two out of the fifty-five senators present voted for it. Attached to a larger bill, the amendment then proceeded quietly and quickly through the House Committee on Ways and Means, the Senate Committee on Finance, and the conference committee, at which point the president signed it into law.

Ever since that time, Medicare runs a program that essentially guarantees access to lifelong regular dialysis to everyone who needs it until they can obtain a transplant, where scarce supply is still an issue. The annual estimated cost of this program today is over $30 billion, accounting for around 7 percent of the Medicare budget, spent on about 1 percent of Medicare patients. The universal, fully subsidized access to one expensive, lifesaving treatment explains the presence of for-profit dialysis centers even in poor neighborhoods, where there are other pressing health care needs that aren't being met, such as for the complications of diabetes, many of which would cost considerably less per person or even in the aggregate.

What separates the funding of universal access to renal dialysis from access to other catastrophic and life-extending health care treatments that have repeatedly failed to win bipartisan congressional support? One element that sets dialysis apart and makes its funding so hard to resist politically is that it is so closely tied to the line dividing life and death. To dramatize the point, and make the case for government funding, Theodore Tsaltas, a Philadelphia doctor who dialyzed himself, testified before the House Committee on Appropriations in 1965. He was featured in an NBC TV documentary that also compared how much the government spent on space exploration. Organized advocates understood that a "show beats a tell," so a patient was dialyzed before the House Committee on Ways and Means in 1971. Within a year, Congress passed the special program. Medicare coverage has never been similarly extended, for example, to people suffering from hemophilia who need blood replacement therapies to survive, despite considerable efforts by their advocates. No public official argues for ending the renal dialysis program today, even while many staunchly advocate cutting Medicaid payments to the states, which support health care for more than seventy million low-income children and adults.

It's hard not to conclude that kidney disease patients, many of whom were middle class, had better advocates and more power at the voting booth in 1972 than millions of poor women, men, and children had then or have today. Just eight years after its passage, the program's cost had quadrupled. Doctors were reporting that dialysis patients were often deeply unhappy, had a suicide rate seven times the national average, and included many chronically ill patients who could afford treatment only for dialysis and not for their other expenses or ailments. The dialysis treatment population skyrocketed because the subsidy for dialysis was so unusually unconditional and patients were not dying from other diseases. By 1980, the dialysis population included, as Gina Kolata reported, "senile patients who are delivered to dialysis centers three times a week from their nursing homes. For some patients, the dialysis machine has become the equivalent of the respirator, sustaining life when hope of regaining health is gone." With universal health care coverage so difficult to achieve in the United States and health care costs escalating, the renal dialysis program remains a unique carve-out in the federal budget.

The life-and-death stakes of funding renal dialysis were clearer than those of many other new treatments that pose a thornier question: What should governments and insurers do about very expensive approved drugs that are intended to extend the lives of a few people when the evidence of benefit isn't totally clear? Insurers increasingly face this question as many new drugs come on the market with questionable or limited benefit for "rare" diseases (defined as affecting fewer than two hundred thousand Americans). Some insurers are balking at covering them. In 2017 the *New York Times* reported that some insurance companies are refusing to pay for the high-cost drug Exondys 51 for Duchenne muscular dystrophy, at least $300,000 a year per child and perhaps as much as five times that. The FDA temporarily approved the drug pending more clinical test results, so at least one insurer considers Exondys 51 to still be "investigational." The FDA's own advisors concluded that the evidence for the drug so far is thin at best. At the same time, children with muscular dystrophy daily undergo irreversible muscle wasting, their desperate parents clutching every possibility to extend their lives. On a conditional basis, the drug company is covering the cost for several well-publicized cases, but that can't go on forever. Does government, in the form of the Medicaid program for low-income people, have an obligation to provide those drugs?

Iron lungs and artificial kidneys are mechanical interventions in basic physiological processes—breathing or cleansing the blood—

and the consequences for life and death are crystal clear. Unlike controversial drugs for rare diseases that extend life but don't lead to a "cure," those seem to many Americans like easy calls, even though both the machines and the drugs are expensive. What they have in common, though, is that the people who are potentially deprived of one or the other are identifiable. There were far fewer ways to learn about polio victims in the 1950s or end-stage kidney disease patients in the early 1970s than about today's patients. Their stories were usually told by journalists, but often not immediately, while today's patients and families have direct access to a far wider range of media, including social media that enable heart-wrenching stories to go viral, sometimes in a matter of minutes. The declining faith in institutions and experts, along with the soaring media capacity to captivate audiences by conveying inaccurate information, also helps rationalize the attitude that everything should be paid for, and without any cost controls, because it just might work—that is, until the bill comes due and the trade-off with other desirable goals becomes clear.

DELIBERATING ABOUT ETHICAL ACCESS

When Congress funded only renal dialysis, it could be criticized for doing too little. It failed to fund universal access to the other health care treatments that people need and should be afforded by right. Less obviously, Congress also could be criticized for doing too much in funding one expensive lifesaving treatment without any built-in cost controls for all individuals regardless of their financial need. The truth is, nearly every society can well afford to provide a decent form of health care to all who need it; whether or not it can muster the political will to do so is another story. The closest any American governmental entity came to endorsing a right to health care was in 1983, when a presidential bioethics commission concluded that "society has an ethical obligation to ensure equitable access to healthcare for all," citing "the special importance of health care," including its role in increasing opportunity. Notably, the commission deliberately avoided the more contentious language of a "right" to health care, because that would imply that someone—by their lights, the "collective American community"—has a duty to provide it. Nonetheless, by avoiding the stronger assertion all those years ago, and especially with that pale reference to the "collective American community," the commission missed a chance to establish a more forceful landmark. Even in the early 1980s, when health care was far less expensive, the commission worried about "rising health care costs and expenditures" and that an equitable system must not be balanced on the backs of the most vulnerable.

Then, as now, for universal health care to be defensible, it must be affordable by both society and the individuals it serves. Libertarianism calls our attention to the need to control government spending, which Congress did not do when it carved out unlimited funding for renal dialysis. As dissenting Utah senator Wallace Bennett put it in 1972, in funding renal dialysis, Congress was drawing upon taxpayers' dollars to fund "Christmas in September." The Christmas present, we would note, was to those who stood to profit from renal dialysis's uncontrolled price. Saving people's lives at no risk to one's own can hardly be considered a luxury or "Christmas present." Bennett also said he was open to compromise and reluctant to discriminate among those suffering from deadly diseases. A more reasonable approach to only funding renal dialysis, he argued, would be to bring forward a "broader health insurance bill" that would insure everyone against catastrophic illness and avoid the blatant unfairness of a single-disease carve-out. A half century later, Congress still has not taken Bennett's prescient point.

When governmental funds are directed to health care in order to save lives, utilitarians call for saving as many lives as possible. No calculation was ever even remotely offered to justify only funding renal dialysis. Senators who spoke in favor of funding the dialysis program conceded this weakness. In reply to Bennett, Senator Russell B. Long, who chaired the Committee on Finance, instead pleaded with his colleagues that the "very unfortunate citizens with chronic renal

failure cannot wait" and called on the next Congress to provide catastrophic health insurance for all Americans. He and an overwhelming majority of his colleagues then passed the buck forward to the
next Congress, which included many of them. Almost a half century
later, Congress is still passing this buck.

Enable everyone to meet their health care needs, control taxation
but not at the expense of people's health and safety, and maximize
social welfare. These precepts of liberalism, libertarianism, and utilitarianism, respectively, provide common reference points in public
debates over the government's role in funding health care, and they
inform critiques of Congress. For skeptics of philosophic perspectives,
there's also simply compassion. But if compassion called for funding
renal dialysis, then why should Congress only fund dialysis and use a
quasi-surreptitious process to pass it through Congress? Why shield
costly and consequential decisions from broader public scrutiny?

Two other major perspectives, deliberative democracy and classical conservatism, illuminate the processes that can best guide governments forward. Deliberative democracy calls upon citizens and
their representatives to deliberate and decide in a way that's publicly
accountable and morally responsible. As "an essential response to
authoritarian populism and post-truth politics," reasons, arguments,
and evidence are offered that try to justify public policies and that
express respect for people across political divides. In politics as in
life, reason-giving alone won't be successful—far from it. Passionate
advocacy and emotional appeals are needed to grab and to hold people's attention. But without offering good reasons, based on sound
evidence, policy makers abdicate their responsibility: public policies
that bind other people demand justification.

Democratic deliberation enables policies to be revised and improved
over time in light of new evidence and argument. This iterative public
process of reciprocal reason-giving aims to craft policies that serve
the common good. While no policy-making process is perfect, and
none can guarantee achieving the common good, democratic deliberation seeks to achieve the common good over time, finding defen-

sible common ground where feasible, and doing so while expressing mutual respect in the middle of ongoing disagreement.

Congress failed to engage in an open, deliberative process when it funded renal dialysis. "The absence of legislative hearings meant that the positions developed were never publicly articulated," one analyst observed. Policy analysis "was deliberately kept at a very low profile" and the issuing of a policy report "was done in an almost surreptitious manner." In how it funded renal dialysis, Congress shielded itself from public pressure to fund a broader health insurance bill that would be more justified by liberal, utilitarian, and deliberative democratic perspectives. The skyrocketing costs of the dialysis program added another obstacle in the way of passing a more universal health insurance bill, despite its greater benefits for the American public. When Congress abdicates its deliberative responsibility with regard to health care, it poorly serves the American public. Yet funding for the dialysis program has never been seriously threatened, perhaps because access to the machines represents life or death within a matter of days.

While deliberative democracy calls for reasoned argument among stakeholders and their representatives in deciding public policies, classical conservatism warns against trusting the powers of human reasoning in seeking rapid large-scale changes in social arrangements, especially through government. Classical conservatives view government as an inherently dangerous necessity, and strongly recommend hedging against large-scale changes in social arrangements, no matter how reasonable they are, especially when these depend upon governmental action. This conservative tradition emanates from the thought of the eighteenth-century Anglo-Irish philosopher and parliamentarian Edmund Burke, and it resonated in the twentieth-century work of the British philosopher Michael Oakeshott. It places a high value on tradition, on what Burke calls "prejudice," as embodied in human institutions wrought from implicit, incremental, and iterative experience. Burke was critical of the French Revolution, perceived as a radical break with traditional political and social institutions, but supportive of the American Revolution, which he regarded as defending institutions that were largely continuous with those of the mother country who, he argued, had rashly provoked the colonies into revolt.

Adapted to the contemporary context, conservatism eschews the idea that there is a natural aristocracy; it values incremental rather than radical change. Conservatives today remain skeptical about rapid, large-scale change according to anyone's preconceived plan. "Change," *New York Times* columnist David Brooks says in homage to Burke, "should be steady, constant and slow. Society has structural problems, but they have to be reformed by working with existing materials, not sweeping them away in a vain hope for instant transformation." Conservatism offers a mixed review of Congress's approach to renal dialysis and health care: criticism of the government for rapidly funding an unprecedented program with a skyrocketing price tag, but relief over its not rapidly enacting universal comprehensive health insurance in one fell swoop.

The checks and balances of American government provide an important structural safeguard against a vulnerability of deliberative democracy: overconfidence in the outcome of reasoned collective decision-making processes. The corresponding blind spot of classical conservatism is complacency with institutionally deep and divisive injustices that many people have long identified and undeservedly endured. Eschewing such complacency, conservatives who consider government a dangerous necessity can still support meeting everyone's need for catastrophic health care coverage (as some conservatives advocated half a century ago). Given that access to catastrophic health insurance has long been recognized as necessary for life itself, a government that enables everyone to afford health care for catastrophic illnesses would make incremental progress that increases social stability and solidarity, rather than the reverse. Half a century ago in the United States, "steady, constant, and slow" progress demanded affordable universal access to catastrophic health insurance. Multiple congresses fell far short of enacting this modest goal that's consistent with common sensibilities, be they conservative or libertarian, liberal or utilitarian.

When values as profound as life, liberty, and opportunity are at stake in access to health care, we also need to question whether modest goals suffice. Who can deny that American history is replete with traditional institutions supporting long-standing injustices—including slavery, disenfranchised women and minorities, laws against miscegenation, and eugenic sterilization laws—which have been upended by social movements rallying around the ideals of equal liberty, opportunity, and justice? "It is of course entirely correct, and a fact confirmed by all historical experience," the social historian Max Weber noted, "that what is possible would never have been achieved if, in this world, people had not repeatedly reached for the impossible." Whether the American people achieve what has seemed impossible only in America, not in other industrialized countries, will depend on the answer to a fundamental question of democratic politics: Will enough people across the country mobilize, organize, fund-raise, and vote for politicians who staunchly support affordable universal health care to overpower the historically more organized, well-funded, and powerful opposition?

AMERICA'S UPHILL BATTLE FOR UNIVERSAL HEALTH CARE

America's failure to provide all its citizens with adequate health insurance remains a fact of our national life. While President Trump frequently promises to provide all Americans with "great" health care, his administration has taken measures that undermine the Affordable Care Act (ACA) without replacing it with something better. One administrative measure taken in 2018 instituted rules that make it easier to sell Americans what is charitably described as "junk insurance": health plans that are too cheap to be true. They exclude pre-existing conditions and cap coverage at a low level, leaving enrollees with unaffordable medical bills when they get seriously ill (something everyone is entitled to be insured against). At the same time, these junk plans draw people away from ACA plans, thereby undermining ACA financing.

Those who are understandably drawn to low-premium health "insurance" to protect themselves and their family because they cannot afford anything else are not to blame for their elected officials' failure of moral leadership. Some of these enrollees will be driven into destitution, and many health systems will have to find ways to compensate for their care, often by raising rates, finding ways to avoid caring for the most expensive uninsured patients, and obtaining support from city and state governments. Thus the health care insurance clock in the United States is turned back. "You'll get such low prices for such great care," President Trump declared in 2017. Political rhetoric is one thing; a cruel hoax is another. The ACA remains under political attack with no substitute in sight, and some of the most vulnerable Americans are unprotected against catastrophic illness. At the same time, more Americans have been signing up for the subsidized insurance that meets ACA standards, demonstrating the law's remarkable resilience under ongoing fire in a hyperpolarized partisan environment.

It is easy to forget that even a program like Medicare, so celebrated today for keeping seniors and their families out of poverty, was *extremely* controversial when first proposed. The term "socialized medicine" has been used for decades by opponents of anything resembling national health insurance. Those watching television one night in 1965 saw the president of the American Medical Association (AMA) sweeping his arm dramatically around an empty auditorium, complaining that this same venue in which President Johnson had spoken for free the previous night was one that his association had to pay for. Then the AMA president lambasted the proposed Medicare program that was likely to be passed through a combination of Johnson's forceful legislative skills—LBJ was notorious for tactics that ranged from exhaustive persuasion to outright bullying—and the reluctance of Congress to block what the recently assassinated President Kennedy would have wanted to see passed. The AMA vehemently opposed the passage of Medicare and also stubbornly refused to recognize that the same forces driving up the costs of medicine were impoverishing many families that were devoted to the care of their elderly relatives, such as unregulated fee-for-service practices that incentivized overtreatment.

As Paul Starr's social history of medicine amply demonstrates, the AMA has been a major force in derailing both earlier and later efforts at more universal coverage than Medicare and Medicaid. During the 1930s New Deal era, the AMA's public attacks on including national health care insurance in social security led President Franklin Delano Roosevelt to back off of it lest the rest of his social security plan otherwise fail. When as part of his Fair Deal in the late 1940s President Harry Truman promoted universal health insurance, the AMA mounted the costliest lobbying campaign ever to oppose it, and disappear it did. Fast forward to the 1990s, when President Clinton proposed a universal health insurance plan and the AMA, while no longer representing a majority of doctors, still exerted its considerable public influence to oppose major parts of the plan that would have expanded coverage and controlled costs. Along with massive opposition by the health insurance industry, the AMA stoked public fears that health care would be rationed in draconian ways and patients would not be able to choose their fee-for-service doctors.

The era that the AMA was defending as recently as the 1990s soon vanished, and the AMA has modified its views about the government's role in health insurance. But the medical leaders of that time were right that opening up the doctor-patient relationship to greater regulation through government insurance would introduce other players into the consulting room, including family members, patient advocates, health care economists, and bioethicists. Today the AMA and many health care leaders accept—perhaps even appreciate—the need for broader consultation.

Many health care providers today also support the expansion of health insurance to more Americans through Medicare and Medicaid. While the AMA's position has moved to approve of expanded coverage of people and their medical conditions (while remaining opposed to a single-payer system), other major players in American

politics have shifted in the polar opposite direction. Generally supporting "access" to the health care that patients need remains a popular position, but a highly ambiguous one: Does access entail (how
much?) subsidized funding (by government and/or employer?) for the
vast majority of Americans who otherwise cannot possibly afford the
costs? Whether and how to make health care universally affordable
has long been a major polarizing issue in American politics.

Besides President Johnson's leadership with members of Congress,
what finally made the establishment of both Medicare and Medicaid possible in 1965 was something that has been sorely lacking
over recent decades especially at the national level: bipartisanship.
The Democratic bill for hospital insurance was combined with elements of a Republican bill for voluntary supplemental health insurance, becoming Parts A and B of Medicare. Medicaid—a federal
matching-funds program that incentivized states to aid Americans
living at or near the poverty line—was packaged to be passed at the
same time. That ingenious "three-layer cake," brokered by the hugely
powerful chairman of the House Committee on Ways and Means
Wilbur Mills, garnered 307 votes in the House of Representatives
including 70 Republicans, with 68 Republicans and 48 Democrats
opposed. In the Senate, it passed 70 to 24, including "yes" votes by
13 Republicans. Seven Democrats and 17 Republicans voted "no."

The rhetoric of socialized medicine continues to resonate strongly
with politicians and citizens who adamantly oppose the mandating
of health insurance or health care entitlements for all. Their identi-
fication of socialized medicine with the overreaching state, however,
is hard to reconcile with the failure of many of the same people to
defend core human freedoms from interference by the state, such as
gay rights, women's rights, civil and religious freedoms for minorities,
and separation of church and state.

Cutting across their ideological differences, however, the vast
majority of older Americans deem the Medicare program incredibly
successful. Surveys indicate that 85 percent of seniors on Medicare
like their plan, a remarkable showing for any government program.

They have both self-regarding and other-regarding reasons to approve. Poverty rates among seniors have plummeted partly because they no longer have to worry about health care costs when they become ill, a huge relief not only to the seniors themselves but also to their families. Healthier and older people are more likely to vote, and older people are a large proportion of the American population, so it has become risky for politicians to threaten Medicare, a "third rail" of American politics (along with social security). A peculiar measure of Medicare's success and the loss of trust in government is that some beneficiaries don't seem to realize it's a government program.

The history of health care reform in the United States teaches us that there is nothing inevitable about achieving universal affordable health care. It is an uphill battle. Attempts at major health care reform over the past century failed under the administrations of Franklin Delano Roosevelt, Harry Truman, Richard Nixon, and Bill Clinton. We learn another lesson from the resistance met by President Barack Obama when, beginning in 2008, he made extending health care coverage to all Americans a priority of his first term. His reform efforts elicited protests that included the vehement plea to "Keep your government hands off my Medicare." Not coincidentally, President Obama's plan did try to assure Americans that the federal government would not be decreasing government benefits. Otherwise it would have been dead on arrival.

Despite an uphill struggle in a highly polarized politics, the Obama administration's health care reform ultimately passed. Far from being perfect from any comprehensive ethical perspective on distributive justice, the plan was a compromise, expanding coverage for millions of uninsured while permitting most but not all Americans who already had health insurance to keep it. (Several million had to switch insurance because it didn't meet the mandated minimal guidelines.) In a highly polarized politics, even this compromise faced resistance within just the liberal Democratic party, where it barely won passage (along with two independent votes). Any "ethically perfect" plan on offer—one that eschewed all compromises—

would certainly have failed. Yet major health care reform passed on party lines that positioned a bitterly opposed Republican party to rally its base around "repeal and replace Obamacare." With little disposition to compromise within its own ranks, the Republicans faced a steep uphill battle to agree upon a replacement.

Conservatism that favors compromise both between and within parties in order to pass legislation was built into American constitutional democracy, famously structured with checks and balances. When politicians are unwilling to compromise, passing legislation is more difficult than blocking it, so the structured default of American politics is inaction, aka gridlock. What's often overlooked is a complementary kind of conservatism built into human psychology: most people react much more strongly to the risk of *losing* something that they perceive as valuable than they do to the prospect of *gaining* the equivalent in value. Losses typically loom about twice as large as equivalent gains. Even people without a competitive nature tend to notice the cars that pass them on the highway more than those that they pass. The renal dialysis subsidy—provided today to about five hundred thousand Americans, many of them middle class—has persisted untouched because a large group of politically powerful Americans would fight fiercely and effectively to keep it.

Especially in American politics, gains are generally harder to achieve than losses are to avert. Add increasing political polarization to this mix, and achieving universal and affordable health care becomes a steeper uphill battle—a steep uphill battle but still a worthy and winnable one. Achieving universal and affordable health care coverage is worthy by the lights of liberalism, Hayekian libertarianism, utilitarianism, and deliberative democratic processes by which citizens can publicly justify to one another meeting everyone's basic health care needs. Conservatism can make the case for an overdue extension of health care coverage to all Americans for the sake of solidarity and social stability. These perspectives, drawing upon different substantive and procedural principles, can converge in support of meeting the health care needs of all individuals within the limits of affordability. To put a human face on these principles is to support all the people who want and need access to affordable health care in their daily lives.

Americans have long been divided and they remain so on whether the federal government has a responsibility to make health care accessible and affordable to all. In 2017 national surveys, for example, the Pew Research Center found that 60 percent of Americans say "the federal government is responsible for ensuring health care coverage for all Americans, while 39% say this is not the government's responsibility." Despite its popularity in opinion polling, ensuring health care coverage for all is still far from an American reality.

A three-to-two margin would be a landslide level of support for any major governmental policy were it not for another fact: national health care reform has been a major epicenter of the political polarization in American two-party politics for a half century or more. The same survey that shows 60 percent of Americans supporting universal health care as a governmental responsibility also reveals striking polarization across party lines: while over 8 of 10 Democrats and Democratic-leaning independents *endorse* this governmental responsibility, over 6 out of 10 Republicans and Republican-leaning independents *oppose* it. Such sharp polarization reinforces our prognosis that until major bipartisan compromise can be reached on health care reform, combining more coverage with greater cost controls, universal and affordable health care in the United States is unlikely to become a reality.

Universal and affordable health care coverage—coupling expanded coverage with controlled costs—will be achieved only if enough citizens reject a system that charges them too high a price for unfair health care and they also mobilize, organize, fundraise, and vote across party lines so that elected officials finally meet the challenge of crafting a comprehensive, twenty-first-century health care system.

Why do we think affordable universal health care is such a worthy cause? For us, it comes down to the fact that health care and public health—from prenatal and postnatal care, clean air and clean water onward—make it possible for everyone to enjoy all the other good things in life. We call health care a human right, because without it we all lack the capacity and the fair equality of opportunity to enjoy everything else in life. For a right to health care to be meaningful, however, it must also be affordable, so we believe people have a right to an *adequate and affordable level* of health care.

Determining what's adequate and affordable is indeed difficult. Should modest health benefits to larger numbers of people, for example, outweigh bigger benefits to smaller numbers, or vice versa? In 1990 the Oregon Health Services Commission made an extensive effort to enable the state to expand its Medicaid coverage for many more low-income citizens. The commission produced an initial draft of the list of treatments to be covered by the state's Medicaid program based on a cost-benefit calculation: "Tooth-capping procedures ended up ranked higher than appendectomies because [of] . . . their having the lower cost-benefit ratio of the two." Counterintuitive examples abounded—thumb-sucking treatment ranked higher than cystic fibrosis or AIDS treatment—with the result being "a public relations disaster."

Simple cost-benefit calculations do not reliably define rights. A right to health care cannot mean that everyone has a right to get their teeth capped but the poor will be out of luck, save for the kindness of strangers, if they need an emergency appendectomy. After the public outcry, the Oregon Medicaid program revised its list and its ranking method so that treating life-threatening ailments outweighed treating more minor benefits to larger numbers of people. It discovered the hard way that a right to health care must cover proven lifesaving treatments and proven early-childhood preventive medicine. It must meet its members' most basic health care needs. And be affordable. But it need not end there.

Democracies cannot avoid the challenge of collectively deciding—often amid heated disagreement and extensive lobbying efforts by interest groups—who should receive how much and what kind of health care. There's no objective formula that can justify bypassing reasonable public deliberation in a democracy. That's what the Oregon Health Services Commission discovered when their first set of priorities relied exclusively on the computer-generated aggregated results of all their data, based on a cost-benefit formula. Principles and the formulae they generate can serve well as guideposts, but they rarely resolve disagreements over who should have a right to what health care and at what cost to whom.

The Oregon commission developed a new ranking system prioritizing those "essential" and "very important" treatments that saved and extended lives. Its new ranking benefited from the input of citizens from a series of community meetings, where citizens emphasized the values of preventive medicine, comfort care, and family planning services. The commission also revised its list after listening to vocal criticism that it undervalued health care for the disabled, and that its community meetings underrepresented the interests of the most vulnerable, both the poor and the disabled. As one member summarized the commission's journey, "Maybe we're not applying science, but we're applying fairness." All voices matter in moving affordable access to health care forward, but giving voice to the most vulnerable members of our society is critical because they pay the highest price for unfair health care.

LESSONS FROM ROMNEYCARE

The revival of some degree of bipartisanship—which has all but vanished from American politics at the national level—is necessary to make significant progress in expanding affordable health care coverage in twenty-first-century America. Bipartisan political compromise in Massachusetts, an overwhelmingly liberal state, made a comprehensive health reform plan possible there in 2006. As incongruous as it seems in light of the Republicans' lambasting of Obamacare less than four years' later, this major move toward universal health care happened under a Republican governor, Mitt Romney, who became the GOP's candidate for president in 2012. "Romneycare" was a cornerstone of his largely popular governorship that launched him to the nomination. That plan, ironically enough, became the model for Obamacare, so it is important to understand some of Romneycare's major elements and outcomes. It was a compromise between those who preferred a single-payer system (with mandated, fully subsidized, and standardized universal coverage) and those who preferred a much more fully market-based system (incentivizing but not mandating coverage and more strictly controlling taxpayer costs).

Why wasn't Romneycare vilified, as Obamacare was? Romneycare relied on shared individual, employer, and government responsibility for insuring all Massachusetts residents, as did Obamacare for insuring all Americans. Both eliminated preexisting conditions as a barrier to receiving health care coverage from private insurers. Both required individuals to attain minimum coverage or pay a tax penalty. Both mandated that, unless they qualify for an exemption, all but the smallest employers provide health insurance to their employees or else pay a fine. Both increased Medicaid benefits and expanded Medicaid coverage to many more low-income Americans. Both created online platforms—called exchanges under Obamacare—where individuals, families, and small employers can choose among a range of private health plans, and both provide many with cost-offsetting subsidies. Both also standardized the benefits in different private plans.

So far, so many similarities. As far as outcomes, in extending health insurance to most Massachusetts residents, Romneycare has been a success. Access to basic health care services increased, and more recipients of health insurance under Romneycare reported receiving good or quality care. Self-assessments report improved physical, mental, and overall health, and mortality data support these self-assessments. By 2010 the state's non-elderly uninsured dropped while the U.S. average increased. (The elderly were already covered by Medicare.) Massachusetts also adopted the expansion of Medicaid offered (but not mandated) by Obamacare, and its uninsured rate fell to the lowest of all fifty states. By comparison, Obamacare's success was more mitigated and continually contested. After its major provisions went into effect (2013–2016), the uninsured rate fell in every state and the overall uninsured rate also dropped significantly. But a significant percentage of Americans continued to be uninsured because many states with high poverty and uninsured rates chose not to opt into the federally subsidized expansion of Medicaid. Its goalpost of extending coverage to all Americans moved closer but was still far from sight.

One key difference is that proportionately more Americans remain uninsured under Obamacare, but that's a likely result of Obamacare's unpopularity rather than a cause. The lack of sufficient cost controls does not differentiate the two plans in favor of Romneycare. Health care costs significantly increased in Massachusetts after the passage of Romneycare. Not surprisingly though, since it expanded coverage to individuals without setting any limits on costs or increases in taxes, producing high health spending and the highest individual insurance costs in the country. In 2012 Massachusetts governor Deval Patrick signed a sweeping bill to limit health care spending to grow no faster than the state's economy; the bill shifted payments away from fees for every service and toward "bundled" payments based on overall patient care. An important lesson of Romneycare: we can't afford to have universal health care and not control costs too.

But the question remains: Why wasn't Romneycare vilified like Obamacare? We know that a vocal minority seized every opportunity to vilify America's first black president, going so far as to incessantly deny the incontrovertible fact of his U.S. birth, questioning his very legitimacy as president. But why did the Affordable Care Act, which provided health insurance to millions more Americans, many of them not Democrats and not in "blue" states, provoke a much broader base of unrelenting, vehement opposition, basically uniting Republicans in opposition (but tellingly not in support of an alternative)? The major difference may seem as obvious as its implications are profound: a bipartisan coalition passed Romneycare and had a vested political interest in supporting its popularity against inevitable opposition. At the national level, the general resistance to bipartisan compromise grew exponentially greater, as did the consequences of no bipartisan support for a major health care reform.

Another major challenge in achieving affordable, universal health care is that in our federal system, states can pursue different goals that result in radically different treatment of their most vulnerable members. To understand the different goals among states is to also appreciate the positive difference that democratic compromise at the state level can make to millions of people's lives. Texas and Mississippi were among the states that refused to accept Medicaid expansion and they had the two highest uninsured rates. Compare Arkansas and West Virginia, similarly majority Republican or "red" states. They also began with high poverty and uninsured rates but within three years decreased their uninsured rates dramatically. West Virginia exemplifies how progress can be made across partisan lines when something as important as people's health is at stake:

> State officials, health care providers and local advocacy groups embraced the Affordable Care Act wholeheartedly—and avoided the word Obamacare. The state didn't just expand Medicaid, but also took extra efforts to identify residents who were likely to be eligible for new insurance, sought them out, and made it easier for them to sign up.

Expanding health insurance succeeded to the extent that it became a bipartisan position in West Virginia politics. Those Republican states, like Arkansas and West Virginia, that compromised by opting into Medicaid expansion successfully decreased their uninsured rates.

The trajectory of Romneycare from coverage to cost control can be a model for national health care coverage when some greater degree of bipartisanship—however unlikely in the short run—returns in America's future. Although very similar in substance, these health care reforms were enacted by tellingly different processes. The most significant fact for understanding the future of universal, affordable health care at the national level: Romneycare was a popular bipartisan compromise, whereas Obamacare passed with not a single Republican crossover vote. Obamacare included increased coverage but unlike Romneycare it also raised taxes and attempted some cost controls. Even if defensible under polarized political circumstances, Obamacare's differences did not make it popular. Precisely the opposite. Also problematic was the fact that, for sound political reasons, the Obama administration had to give up a "public option" early in negotiations with a Republican Congress. That proposal would have created a government insurance agency to compete with private plans, bringing down premiums. It failed to pass due to intense lobbying by the health insurance companies, using the old cliché of socialized medicine as cover. Losing the public option somewhat deflated enthusiasm for Obamacare on the left. To make matters worse, the federal government bungled and delayed the rollout of its central website, Healthcare.gov, an essential aid intended to enroll tens of millions of Americans who otherwise would remain uninsured. Although a bumpy rollout of the website didn't help, bugs in a complicated online system are not unique to government and are common in the private sector. The rollout was a convenient target.

Polls of the American public have rarely shown bare majority support for Obamacare, and not even that for any proposed alternative in the long Republican campaign to repeal and replace it. When it comes to passing major legislation that has staying power by gaining popular support over time, the best bet in American politics is not pretty by liberal, libertarian, or utilitarian lights: it's bipartisan compromise. But just wishing for more bipartisanship is naïve, so Americans need to ask ourselves: What will really happen if more voters across party lines do not mobilize, organize, and support candidates willing to advance a common good? The most likely outcome is political stalemate; in this case, the steep price is leaving millions of our fellow Americans without affordable health care.

PROGRESS TOWARD A COMMON GOOD

What might it realistically take to make progress toward the common good of universal affordable health care? Multiple obstacles to affordability remain. Fee-for-service practices where medical services are paid for separately, for example, create incentives to give more tests and treatments, not only adding more costs but also leading to overtreatment and more burdens for patients. Sometimes those burdens lead to a cascade of interventions like overprescribed drugs and unnecessary surgeries that carry their own risks to the patient's health. At the other extreme, early health maintenance organizations experimented with "capitation," paying a medical practice a lump sum per patient. But capitation creates incentives for undertreatment. Bundled payments are a compromise that pays for expected episodes of medical care based on expected needs of the patient.

What progress is possible in a hyperpartisan, polarized political system? Not enough, to be sure. That's why the single greatest harbinger for progress in addressing the high cost of unfair health care in America will be more citizens educating one another, mobilizing, registering, and voting for positive change. But even now we can take positive steps that are critical to every American's health and well-being. One reform that we suggest is part and parcel of informed consent to health care: patients should know what they and their insurers are paying for. A maddening fact of life in American health care is that it is so difficult to understand a medical bill. Despite the evolving notions about patients' rights to truth and information, medical billing remains an outlier. Not only are medical bills rife with abbreviations and codes that require a veritable Rosetta Stone to interpret, they are often laced with errors about (and charges for) services that weren't rendered. There are many ethically challenging issues in health care, but this isn't one of them. As one physician-journalist has written, patients have "the right to an itemized bill in plain English."

Long before billing, the lack of price accountability runs deep in the process of providing health care. Patients have little if any clarity about the prices of elective procedures, which should be provided in advance. Informed consent to health care must mean telling patients beforehand about the costs of any elective procedures, but far from being routinely practiced, it's typically neglected and unenforced. Other reasonable expectations for patients and their families include no surprise billing; that their "provider" network be stable enough to prevent sudden out-of-network charges; and that they be made aware of conflicts of interest that could influence the way they are treated, like the way the hospital expects the doctor to generate revenue.

Greater price accountability and transparency is a start that's likely to generate greater public pressure in the direction of controlling costs for patients, which in turn will provide greater access to health care. But it's only a start. Other initiatives, suggested by the surgeon-scholar Atul Gawande, would increase the incentives for responsible treatment and pricing. Using their positive power, the media can shine a spotlight on local health care systems that are overtesting and overtreating patients with demonstrably bad results, in striking comparison with those producing better results at lower costs to both patients and the public. In comparing health care systems in El Paso, Texas, with McAllen, Texas, Gawande reveals this striking "cost conundrum": "Unnecessary care often crowds out necessary care, particularly when necessary care is less remunerative." But what to do about this when governments won't act to control costs at the macro level? Try incentive systems at the local level, Gawande suggests. Local health care systems can improve care while they cut down on costs by sharing their savings with doctors. Insurance companies can similarly incentivize hospitals, but the incentives must be designed with health outcome measures that guard against the equally dangerous side effect of undertreatment.

Progress toward universal affordable access to health care requires much more. To make health insurance financially viable for private or public insurers, more and less healthy populations must be pooled and treatment costs must be controlled. This is what enables the less healthy—whatever their ideology—to afford their health care today, and the healthier among us today to afford it when our health unexpectedly takes a turn for the worse in the future.

Modern health care is an expensive necessity; costs must be controlled and access must be increased. A critical question is whether cost controls will happen in a publicly accountable way. Drug pricing is an example. In recent decades, many drug prices have skyrocketed, and drug costs account for a significant part of the most recent rise in health care costs. If left uncontrolled, universal health care becomes increasingly difficult if not impossible for even an affluent society to afford. As several experts on the U.S. system point out, "the United States is distinct in that it offers strong drug patent protections and limits the ability of public and private payers to appraise new drugs and bargain effectively for lower prices."

Patent protections fuel innovation, but they needn't do so at the expense of access if the largest payers are empowered to appraise all drugs and negotiate lower prices. Given that the federal government is the single largest payer, empowering Medicare to control costs would be a major step forward. Without this capacity to negotiate prices based on cost-effectiveness and other common metrics of value, private health insurers often insist on paying for the least expensive drug even if a more expensive one significantly improves the patient's life. New drugs and treatments that can bring dramatic improvements in patient care will be unaffordable if the costs of ineffective and less effective drugs and treatments are not reviewed and controlled. The magnitude and significance of the cost-control, limited accessibility problem faced by the United States today is huge. We will squander the means of enabling all people to live healthier lives if we don't muster our collective will to control costs.

Pharmaceuticals are only part of the problem, but higher drug prices are the single biggest factor—according to recent studies—that accounts for the greater cost per person of health care in the United States compared to ten other high-income countries (with higher life expectancies than the United States). The differences are glaring: Americans annually spend an average of $1,443 per person on drugs compared to Germany's average of $667 per person, and an average of $749 per person for all eleven affluent countries. These differences are driven primarily by price, not volume of use, making it all the more possible and desirable that the American government—as the single biggest drug funder through Medicare and Medicaid—take steps to control their costs.

Why are cost controls so important? Rather than count all the ways, we'd do well to focus our attention on the unmet health care needs of millions of Americans and on the other unmet needs, such as public education, primarily funded out of state budgets that have been starved over recent years because of escalating Medicaid and other health care costs. As physician-ethicist Ezekiel Emanuel and others have pointed out, Medicaid now accounts for 29 percent of state budgets, a rise of almost 10 percent over just the past decade, while state spending on public education has plummeted.

This trend of escalating health care costs is a long one, and it negatively impacts *all* Americans, those who are well covered by health care insurance (with rates that have continued to rise faster than average incomes) and even more so for the millions who are not adequately insured. Since 1980 America's spending on health care has soared but life expectancy has dipped below that of other developed countries. These conditions have created systematic distortions in our health care system that go well beyond dollars—they shorten lives. A major reason is that the United States spends less on those low on the socioeconomic ladder—the very people, including many children, who are most vulnerable and could benefit the most from improved access to health care. The lack of affordable access to health care, including adequate public health and mental health care, for children and low-income individuals is unfair. And it's also costly. Poor prenatal and postnatal care, lead paint poisoning, polluted drinking water, emergency room visits, and other gross inefficiencies in addressing the health care needs—not just wants—of America's most vulnerable members costs the United States far more than it saves, no matter how costs are reasonably calculated.

Yet another major consequence of health care cost escalation is the starving of public education, which also harms the most vulnerable along with middle-income Americans. As much as Americans value the freedom to choose, that freedom of choice has a collective compo-nent that we neglect at enormous ethical and practical peril: together we can all afford the health care we will need only by agreeing to pool risks, to control costs, and to subsidize the costs of coverage when most of us are still healthy. Otherwise Americans face an indefinitely long future of an unsustainably expensive and unfair system.

Six

FORAGING
FOR ETHICS

Behind the escalating cost of health care and our failure to design a system that is fair, efficient, and humane lies one of the most elemental facts of the human condition: scarcity. There is never enough for everything that people need. Or is there? No less a philosopher than Mick Jagger makes a point of distinguishing between "wants" and "needs," famously singing that "you can't always get what you want, but if you try sometimes you might find, you get what you need." Human beings are well designed to forage for what they need. Many neuroscientists think that foraging for scarce food sources was a key part of the development of human society for mutual aid and of the evolution of the human brain. Our ancestors foraged for sweet and fatty things, tastes that purveyors of fast food call "mouthfeel." Those foods contain nutrients necessary for survival and also give the brain a rewarding shot of dopamine. But the hunter-gatherers had to expend a lot of energy on foraging because those sweet and fatty foods were scarce. Some of the sources were hard to kill and could eat us before we could eat them.

In the modern world, we have plenty of easily accessible sweet and fatty items in our environment but the foraging impulse has not been turned off, which partly explains the obesity epidemic and why people in low-income countries tend to gain too much weight once they have plentiful access to high-fat foods. Our brain's prefrontal cortex—the slow-developing site of longer-range decision making and planning—is just about the only part of our entire system that can distinguish between wants and needs, and it's easily overwhelmed by our foraging and feeding impulses.

The distinction between wants and needs in modern health care is important but in practice it's often difficult to apply. Modern advertising is especially adept at convincing us that our needs include pretty much everything on offer in the health care marketplace, including the latest lifestyle drug for a new, improved treatment for male-pattern baldness. And when we can specify certain clear needs, such as clean water or lifesaving organ transplants, even if underrepresented minorities and other low-income Americans try very hard, they often don't get what they need. Meanwhile, some of us may be overtreated, especially celebrities, by being able to insist upon and pay for a cascade of treatments that might do harm delivered by physicians reluctant to say no. Like ordering too many Big Macs, foraging for health care just because it feels good is often a bad idea.

Mostly, though, rather than overproviding the health care that most people need, the United States doesn't provide enough, starting with public health interventions. Especially when it comes to expensive medicine, it turns out that we only get what we need if the health care system has made it accessible and affordable to us. The decisions that have shaped the American health care system often yield inconsistent and inequitable results, like the unique access to kidney dialysis we discussed in the previous chapter while millions of low- and middle-income Americans in need of care for diabetes or hospice or mental illness are left without adequate insurance coverage. It's not unusual for these results to be blatantly unfair, as when a wealthy patient in need of a transplant is permitted to register on several waiting lists for a lifesaving organ. We're not saying that it's always easy to identify unfairness in a health care system, let alone correct it. But the high stakes put the onus on democratic citizens and our government as trustees of the common good to help all people get at least the health care they clearly need.

RATIONING AND SCARCITY

Rationing and scarcity are two interlocking concepts. When a desirable good or service is scarce, it is rationed. Scarcity is sometimes natural, like precious metals or transplantable human organs, but in medical ethics the problem usually involves artificial scarcity, understood as the collective result of many decisions that yield situations that might have been unintended and even unpredictable. A familiar example is the fact that some lifesaving medical products might be manufactured at only one facility, so if that factory goes off-line, it triggers a crisis of scarcity. Rationing is far more common than Americans ordinarily appreciate because it is more often implicit than explicit.

Economists point out that pricing is a form of rationing because it's a way of allocating something desirable when there's not enough for everybody. There are explicit rationing schemes like a lottery or first come, first served. In medical ethics, battlefield triage is the paradigmatic rationing scheme. In a classic triage system, benefit to the collective is prioritized over efforts to benefit individuals. Out of a group of injured soldiers, if not all can be attended to at once, those who can survive without immediate treatment are placed in one category and those unlikely to survive even with treatment are placed in another, so that treatment is provided to those likely to survive and benefit from treatment now. The point is to return as many fighters to the field as is possible under the circumstances. Although triage originated in a military context, in the civilian world it may be a default whenever an emergency medical team can't care for all patients at once, or when the surge capacity of hospitals is exceeded, as in a horrific accident or due to an epidemic. The collective benefit standard leads to some results that are not usually found in health care systems that are based mainly on the prospect of individual benefit, such as the sudden arrival at the field hospital of the general officer who, though less likely to perish than the private she just arrived with, is more important to the war effort. In epidemics where there's a shortage of a vaccine, say, the health care worker is prioritized as a "force multiplier" over others who are also in need but less critical to managing the crisis.

But the classic battlefield triage model and other extreme emergencies like pandemics are poor guides to dealing with scarce and expensive health care resources in the everyday world. On the battlefield the norm is overwhelming deference to collective benefit as determined by authoritative decision makers. Not so in everyday life over the past half century in the United States, as patients have become self-authorizing consumers of health care, employing an enormously complex, quasi-market system that cannot be addressed by means of a simplified priority ordering like triage. To make matters even more complicated, health care costs have rapidly risen, patients have demanded and exercised more voice in their own treatment, and more science-based medicine has delivered and continues to promise new treatments for patients with varying probabilities of success.

One result of these developments has been pressure by patients directly on health care practitioners and indirectly on institutions to provide these goods. The anticipated costs and potential revenues of new treatments have generated countervailing pressures on governments, sometimes highly organized and amply funded by pharmaceuticals and other business interests, not to raise taxes or to control costs at the expense of private-sector profits. In this environment, wants and needs may seem hopelessly entangled.

Amplified by social media and the rising value of self-determination, the patient's voice has especially increased pressure on government to provide greater access to all life-extending drugs and treatments. Often those demands are unaccompanied by a correspondingly strong willingness of *either* institutions *or* individuals to pay for them or to control their costs. Growing numbers of patients are in effect consumers who pay only indirectly for their health care through insurance premiums and taxes, are insulated from actual costs, and are not in a position to assess a test or treatment for safety and efficacy (until it's too late). As the economist Kenneth Arrow originally observed in the 1960s, competitive markets in health care are inevitably inefficient, and over the ensuing decades the costs of this inefficiency have only skyrocketed. Absent any public evaluation of a treatment's cost-effectiveness, the U.S. health care market structure further propels more voices demanding greater access to more newly discovered treatments. Who is willing to be the first to decline a new treatment that we are told is "pathbreaking" or "cutting edge"? In the short term, some sorely needed reforms would both help to reduce drug prices and make the resulting costs clearer, educating health care consumers about the actual value of the services they receive.

For a start, medical bills should be required to itemize charges in clear language, and states should be allowed to negotiate rates for drugs. Congress also should take steps to control exorbitant drug pricing by manufacturers that hold exclusive patents. Excessively long patent protections (not patent protections per se, which are necessary) enable these producers to block healthy market competition when the terms of those patents outlive their usefulness as incentives to innovation. Patents for the new kinds of drugs produced through biological mechanisms—among the most sought after and expensive drugs on the market—create novel challenges that must be addressed. The biological mechanism itself is patentable, leaving open the question of what alternative drugs should and should not be precluded by their patents. Their prices must be made affordable to those who can benefit most from their use. Meanwhile, Medicare should be authorized to negotiate the prices charged for prescription medicines sold to people not in hospital care. Much more consequential will be what happens when our health care system is restructured to incentivize the research and development of what's most cost-effective, as we discuss in chapter 5. Flying cars haven't happened for a reason, and it's not because they can't be made. Hard questions need to be asked about the effectiveness compared with the cost of new drugs, and financial incentives built into health care development and delivery so that the market actually rewards the most effective and affordable options.

EVIDENCE MATTERS

Scarcity is an ironic triumph of modern medical science. Had modern science never perfected organ transplants or discovered the immuno-suppressive drug that made living with them possible, there would never be an organ shortage. The scarcity of dialysis machines created a crisis demanding some form of rationing that lasted over a decade, but then it ended with the ESRD (end-stage renal disease) program that provided dialysis to all in need. There are good reasons for the demand to reduce the artificial scarcities inherent in expensive health care: it means more of the good stuff we have come to expect from the medical science. How could we not want more? The rapid pace of medical progress since World War II has been so remarkable that it virtually beckons to us to insist on more. Polio vaccines made iron lungs a thing of the past. The "magic bullet" called penicillin and other antibiotics are now widely available, rendering age-old scourges like syphilis and other once-deadly infections now matters of routine medical treatment. Antibiotics have become so widely available that their overprescription, overuse, and misuse have created widespread bacterial resistance to antibiotics. The Centers for Disease Control and Prevention (CDC) now calls antibiotic resistance "one of the world's most pressing public health problems." It was easy to be lulled into false confidence, thinking that the era of infectious disease was over and all that Americans needed was to be given ready access to every available health care product and service that each person wanted.

In the 1950s another important set of drugs rapidly came into enormous demand: the birth control pill. Most new drugs were designed to save lives or to prevent or manage disease. Birth control was instantly desirable for equally compelling reasons. In 1960 the first pill specifically for birth control was approved by the Food and Drug Administration (FDA), sending a message to women that mod-ern medicine could provide previously only imaginable opportunities for control over their bodies. Hard as it might be to believe today, married couples didn't even have a legally recognized right to use ordinary contraception until a 1965 Supreme Court decision in the case of *Griswold v. Connecticut. Griswold* became a critical building block in the ever-more controversial 1973 case of *Roe v. Wade*, when the Supreme Court found that the constitutional right to privacy included a woman's right to abortion.

Yet just as Americans were getting adjusted to the idea that it was imperative to make sure lifesaving medicine was available to all who needed it and that a pill could help empower women to control their own lives by more easily and effectively separating sex from reproduction, they were also finding out that too much medicine could be catastrophic. In 1962, only a few months before Shana Alexander's *Life* magazine article about the Swedish Hospital committee making life-or-death decisions, the magazine's readers suddenly saw pictures of babies who were perfect in every way save one: their arms or legs were often severely deformed. The editors of popular publications like *Life* that made their way into people's homes deemed it best not to include certain still more disturbing malformations among their illustrations.

Thalidomide was marketed as a sedative in the late 1950s, often as an anti-nausea medicine for pregnant women, mostly in West Germany but also elsewhere in continental Europe, Great Britain, Canada, and the Middle East. It was *never* approved for sale in the United States (though in an odd twist it was later licensed for the treatment of certain cancers) because an FDA officer named Frances Kelsey was suspicious. An immigrant from Canada to the Midwest, Kelsey received her doctorate in pharmacology and medical degree from the University of Chicago, taught there and at the University of South Dakota, and practiced medicine, becoming a naturalized citizen in 1956. In her attempts to find a synthetic cure for malaria, Kelsey learned that some drugs can pass through the placental barrier. In 1960, already a pioneer as an accomplished female physician, she had just taken a new job at the FDA when an application for a license to market thalidomide landed on her desk. Thalidomide had been marketed in Canada and forty-five other countries, but Kelsey demanded more information from the manufacturer, the William S. Merrell Company in Cincinnati. The company went over Kelsey's head, complaining about her stubbornness and calling her—among other things—"a fussy, stubborn, unreasonable bureaucrat." But Kelsey persisted, and by 1961 there was evidence that thalidomide had caused birth defects in thousands of babies. Vindicated, Kelsey received all manner of recognitions, including a medal from President Kennedy, and is an icon of the drug safety world.

Although the toxic effects of thalidomide on fetuses weren't discovered in a clinical trial, the public reaction was so intense that in 1962 Congress unanimously gave the FDA new powers to assess not only the toxicity but also the efficacy of new drugs prior to approval. New protections for people against medical conflicts of interest also included requirements to report adverse reactions and to obtain informed consent from patients to participate in clinical studies. The U.S. drug regulatory system quickly became a global model. It protects against both the kinds of injuries endured by the children exposed to thalidomide and also helps to prevent exploitation of those who are seriously ill; there's enough of that already. Over the years, the system also has had to strike a balance between these protections and giving terminally ill patients who have exhausted all standard treatments special access to experimental drugs. Yet, just as many Americans have forgotten (or never known) what life was like before vaccines, many have become inured to the importance of these protections.

RIGHT TO TRY?

In a way, we have learned the lessons of modern medical science too well: demand it and it will come. There is a kind of collective frustration when government tells us to cool our heels in our demands for new stuff, that it knows better than we do what will satisfy our health care needs, even if we are seriously ill. A movement that threatens to undermine the FDA's role in protecting the American public succeeded in 2018 in passing a federal law under the misleading name of "right to try." (Most states already had such a law on the books.) Encouraged and enabled by an antigovernment atmosphere that was further stimulated by the Trump campaign, "right-to-try" advocates object not only to the paperwork involved but to the very notion that government should have a role in these decisions.

Opponents of the federal and state right-to-try laws note that in the history of drug testing, some treatments that were promising before they were carefully tested have proven both disappointing and harmful, potentially worsening the end of patients' lives. Open access to medications that have not gone through rigorous clinical trials might also make it more difficult to gain sufficient enrollment for those studies (which generally must involve the chance that a patient will not get the experimental medicine), with the result that some drugs would be widely used without evidence of their efficacy. An example of a treatment that was widely assumed to be effective was bone marrow transplantation for women with breast cancer, which was widely adopted in the 1980s but was proven to be useless in clinical trials. One cancer researcher has written that "more than 30,000 women in the United States with breast cancer received bone marrow transplants between 1985 and 1998, at the cost of millions of dollars, considerable adverse effects, and treatment-related mortality rates of 3 to 15%." Evidence matters.

One principle that everyone should be able to agree on is that when evidence for a treatment is available, whoever has paid for it, that information should be widely available to doctors and patients. Yet in 2018 the Trump administration shut down an online database—the National Guideline Clearinghouse—that was set up in the 1990s to do just that. The Agency for Healthcare Research and Quality, which maintains the information connecting science to medical practice, has been on life support for years. Inefficiency and unfairness are the mildest possible terms for shutting down a reliable public resource in order to save $1.2 million a year in a country that spends $3.5 trillion dollars on health care. This shutdown seriously exacerbates the risks to consumers created by touting a right to try without supporting evidence of effectiveness.

One point that the right-to-try advocates get right is that a properly functioning regulatory system does create a form of artificial scarcity, but the scarcity in question in this case is that of a drug or device with an unproven benefit and potential for exploiting false hopes. There is an irony in the way that the principle of respect for patient autonomy has been stood on its head by right-to-try laws. The principle has been distorted so as to include the right to demand an unproven treatment. Granted that there is a universal desire for access to effective drugs, especially in the face of a terminal illness, but there is not a corresponding willingness to wait for the evidence or pay for the added cost of reliable research. In any case, these laws should really be called "right to ask" for experimental medication because drug companies are not required to participate. And the FDA is not out of the loop yet, despite the shortsighted wishes of many antigovernment advocates, because it has the authority to decide when a drug is safe enough to qualify for a right-to-try claim.

The right-to-try movement is in many ways a continuation of a debate that has been going on ever since the FDA was granted expanded powers following the thalidomide scandal. For about twenty years, there was no written policy about access to "investigational" drugs that are not approved but might benefit an individual patient, so in essence doctors just called to the agency to request a drug for a patient. That process was too random. In the 1980s efforts to formalize the system ran headlong into the HIV/AIDS epidemic, which created an emergency that pitted AIDS activists who insisted on the need for greater access against the agency that was responsible for drug safety. One innovation in the 1990s was a "parallel track" that made some drugs available to people with AIDS who had exhausted all their other options, even without evidence of effectiveness.

Government agencies are not known for the rapidity of their response to the public, and as we have seen, some have contributed their share to losing the public's confidence and trust. However, in this instance the FDA responded with alternative pathways for access to experimental medication. Starting in 1987 the FDA has used a "treatment IND" (investigational new drug) mechanism that makes promising drugs available to people with serious or life-threatening diseases if the risks are justifiable and there is no alternative therapy for those patients, the program widely known as "compassionate use." (The FDA has several different categories of expanded access protocols; we don't summarize them all here.) As painful and fitful as the process has been, adjustments and improvements in rules about access to drugs have been made since thalidomide and can still be made, speeding up bureaucratic processes with gains rather than losses for patient health. Applications for compassionate use for those who don't qualify for a clinical trial are virtually all granted within a few days, rendering right-to-try applications redundant.

In themselves, right-to-try laws are innocuous. But they are also the "canary in the coal mine," with potentially dangerous implications for our world-leading regulatory system. All regulation, including that for medical products, creates an intentional form of artificial scarcity, one aimed at protecting the public from unscrupulous "snake oil" salespeople, especially cruel at the end of life. Liberals and libertarians alike can strongly support regulations that are carefully targeted to prevent fraudulent marketing. The libertarian party platform states that "fraud must be banished from human relationships" and supports "the prohibition of . . . fraud, and misrepresentation."

Fraudulent marketing isn't free marketing. Libertarians may prefer warning labels and consumer education to prohibitions. But a distinctively troubling set of problems accompanies a "warnings only" approach to dangerous drugs and other medical treatments. A free market in dangerous or fraudulent drugs, accompanied only by warning labels and education, not only offers predictably inadequate protection against profit-seeking manipulation of consumers through advertising. It also fails to offer any protection against simple misunderstandings of what a label says, or the all-too-human failure to read the label before ingesting. Marketing something as a therapeutic drug that isn't safe and effective is inherently dangerous, in addition to being fraudulent, because of the potentially dire consequences for defrauded consumers.

These drugs are not taken for pleasure, with a warning that they are bad for your health. They are marketed and taken for health. Dire consequences—as in the case of thalidomide—run precisely counter to their primary purpose. This problem makes stronger regulations, beyond warning labels, acceptable to most people and most ethical perspectives, including some strong interpretations of libertarianism. While government is called upon to subsidize drugs that satisfy health care needs, it's not supposed to subsidize dangerous or futile consumer desires or behaviors. In contrast to government action designed to address the undersupply of iron lungs and dialysis machines *after* they have been deemed safe and effective, drug and device regulation aims to ensure that pharmaceuticals are safe and effective *before* being marketed. These are different senses in which access is limited to health care goods and services that many people may want.

IN THE WEEDS

Overregulation is every bit as bad as underregulation. The decades-long struggle to legalize medical cannabis—aka medical marijuana—is a fascinating example not only of the perils and irrationalities of excessive regulation but also of the creation of scarcity amid plenty. There is no shortage of marijuana but there is a shortage both of cannabis for medical research and a legal system that facilitates the research. The National Institute on Drug Abuse (NIDA) historically oversaw a monopoly on the cannabis grown for medical research. It allowed only one institution, the University of Mississippi, to produce cannabis for federally approved studies, limiting scientific access to a tiny fraction of the hundreds, if not thousands, of cannabis strains available, each of which has a unique cannabinoid profile and potentially a different therapeutic "entourage" effect. For decades, even after successfully braving the especially onerous combination of Drug Enforcement Administration (DEA), FDA, NIDA, and Public Health Service (PHS) reviews, researchers could still wait over a year to receive "research-grade" cannabis, only to find it contaminated by mold or of inferior potency. The tide began to turn in 2015 when the Obama administration did away with the duplicative PHS review. The next year, the DEA allowed more facilities to apply to grow cannabis for medical research, but as we write, no applications have yet been approved, and the DEA has no timeline for acting.

Spurred by the demands of their citizens and the regulatory gridlock undermining the possibility of progress on medical cannabis research and policy, states began to circumvent the federal imbroglio. In 1996 California became the first state to legalize medical cannabis. Two decades later and still without FDA approval, dozens of U.S. states and territories had determined that cannabis is medicine for conditions like pain, epilepsy, and PTSD (posttraumatic stress disorder). Strikingly, in 2017, the National Academies of Sciences, Engineering, and Medicine "found conclusive or substantial evidence . . . for benefit from cannabis or cannabinoids" for such common and debilitating ailments as chronic pain, chemotherapy side effects, and spasticity resulting from multiple sclerosis, and moderate or limited evidence of its effectiveness for a variety of other conditions. Although the FDA has approved several cannabinoid drugs, the agency has not approved medical cannabis as safe or effective for the treatment of any medical indication. Lacking FDA approval, health insurance generally does not cover it, state laws conflict with one another and with a strict federal law, crossing state lines with cannabis remains a federal crime (even from one legal state to another), and employment drug testing for cannabis poses a risk to users.

The contemporary patients' rights movement to legalize medical cannabis in the United States highlights the tension between the interests of patients with unmet medical needs and the barriers erected by regulatory processes to ensure a medication's safety and effectiveness. An online citizen-science movement has recorded and compared tens of thousands of user experiences of many genetic strains of cannabis, empowering patients to better understand what kind of medical cannabis might work for them safely and effectively, how to consume it, and what side effects to watch for. These issues, in our view, are ripe for resolution. Not only is the federal law anomalous, it's likely unsustainable as long as the evidence and public opinion together mount in favor of permitting systematic research on medical cannabis.

SCARCITY AND ORGAN TRANSPLANTS

As transplants have become practical for many end-state kidney disease patients over the years, though still requiring them to take powerful drugs to suppress their immune systems, dialysis has been thought of as a temporary bridge to transplant. Sadly, the artificial scarcity of dialysis machines that was resolved in the 1970s has been replaced by an enormous shortage of transplantable kidneys. The kidney shortage is both natural—because living donors can spare only one—and artificial—because societies have failed to find ways to convince enough healthy people to donate their spare kidneys to meet the dire demand. In spite of aggressive efforts to promote kidney donation, thousands of Americans still die every year while on waiting lists for cadaver organs or for a living donor. One advantage that patients in need of a kidney have over those who need other organs is that nature has given us two and normally we only need one, so sufficient donation from a living human being is, by nature, possible to cover everyone in need. But human compassion has yet to rise to meet this worthy challenge. The same is true for livers as only a portion of the liver, the liver lobe, is needed for transplant and the rest of the organ grows back in the donor, though a whole liver from a dead donor may also be transplanted.

For other solid organs, like hearts, the only option so far is an organ from a cadaver. Heart transplants have become a common procedure but only after a rocky and enormously controversial start in 1967, when a South African surgeon named Christiaan Barnard transplanted a human heart into the chest of fifty-five-year-old Louis Washkansky. The heart came from Denise Darvall, who had been severely injured in a car accident. Dying of his heart disease, Washkansky agreed to the first-ever such transplant with what Barnard estimated was about an 80 percent chance of surviving. The story made huge international headlines and riveted the world. Unfortunately, Washkansky succumbed after only eighteen days due to complications from the immunosuppressant drugs. Nonetheless, the handsome, forty-five-year old Barnard instantly became an international celebrity, which he clearly relished. As to the ethics of the operation, Barnard showed no hesitation: "For a dying man it is not a difficult decision . . . because he knows he is at the end. If a lion chases you to the bank of a river filled with crocodiles, you will leap into the water convinced you have a chance to swim to the other side. But you would never accept such odds if there were no lion."

Lion analogies aside, across the world today only five thousand heart transplants are performed every year. An estimated fifty thousand people are eligible candidates for heart transplantation. The availability of suitable hearts from dead donors for transplant depends to a great extent on the timing. In general, the closer the "harvesting" of the organ is to the actual transplant, the greater the chances for success. It is especially important that the organ is freshly perfused by oxygenated blood. The ethical concept that makes that possible is the "dead donor" rule. Though it might seem somewhat technical, it's important to note exactly what the rule says:

> An individual who has sustained either (1) irreversible cessation of circulatory and respiratory functions, or (2) irreversible cessation of all functions of the entire brain, including the brain stem, is dead. A determination of death must be made in accordance with accepted medical standards.

In other words, the second part of the rule states that organs cannot be taken before the donor's death, but as long as the "person" is dead, death can be determined while the person's body is still alive. For that to happen, the person must be brain dead, though their heart and lungs are still working. An accurate determination that a person's brain is dead means that the person is dead even though other systems may still function. Brain death is now medicine's standard definition of death. It was made a matter of law under the Uniform Determination of Death Act (UDDA), which is now essentially the same in all fifty states and the District of Columbia. Among the most consequential definitions of modern medicine, the brain death standard is inextricably bound up with ethics in at least two ways: first, it asserts that when our brains are dead, we as persons are dead; and second, as a result of this standard, it becomes morally acceptable to take an organ from a brain-dead person to save the life of someone who needs the organ, provided the organ is still working well. Because a major sector of lifesaving medicine depends on these two judgments, and controversy continues to revolve around them, we must recognize their ethical, rather than purely empirical, status.

An ad hoc 1968 Harvard committee was the source of this new standard for death. The committee recognized that the ancient and traditional ways of determining when someone had died, based on hearts and lungs that no longer functioned, were no longer the last word. Neuroscientists had come to understand that the brain operates as the central coordinating system for all bodily processes and without it the body cannot survive long before organs fail and tissues begin to break down. There were also new ways to measure electrical activity in the brain to determine that it had ceased operating. These and other factors contributed to the Harvard committee's conclusion that brain death is death. The brain death standard was propounded just as bioethics was emerging as a field and quickly became closely identified with it as a core premise of modern bioethics.

Crucially, in creating the brain death standard, the committee also intended to ameliorate the natural scarcity of precious human organs for transplant by reducing the prospect of controversy about obtaining organs. Henry Beecher, a professor of anesthesiology, was the chair of the Harvard committee and one of the most colorful and influential characters not only in the history of bioethics but also in the history of medicine in the twentieth century. During World War II, he was stationed at the front in battlegrounds like the Anzio beachhead where he treated young soldiers with horrid injuries. Yet often the soldiers seemed not to suffer from the great pain that would be expected with such severe injuries. Beecher came to appreciate that the mind has a remarkable capacity to modulate the experience of pain. In 1955 he expressed this insight in a famous paper on "The Powerful Placebo." Beecher didn't discover the "placebo effect" but he appreciated its potential more than many others did.

The insight about the placebo effect impressed Beecher with the key role that the brain plays in the nature of experience. When he chaired the Harvard brain death committee, he was more than prepared to take a certain moral and philosophical position on the brain: when it dies, the patient dies. But over the years, doubts about the either-or nature of brain death have grown as new technologies for measuring brain activity have been developed. Like the diagnosis of a vegetative state, the condition about which so much was learned in the landmark case of Karen Ann Quinlan, the diagnosis of brain death is a clinical judgment, though it can be supported by various tests such as an angiography and an EEG (electroencephalography).

In at least one highly publicized California case, a thirteen-year-old African American girl named Jahi McMath remained alive for five years after being diagnosed as dead by brain criteria. Her family had insisted that on religious grounds she should continue to be treated. Many African Americans also have reason to suspect that they are at risk of being undertreated, and worse still at risk of being treated as a means only—for example, as sources of organs for transplant and not as patients for whom doctors will go all out to extend their lives—as they will for other patients. Despite predictions that her body would gradually deteriorate, Jahi's family finally succeeded in having her moved to New Jersey, one of only two states in the United States where religious exceptions to brain death are recognized.

Complicating the picture, neurologists have found that some people who might be diagnosed as in vegetative states are actually misdiagnosed, as modern brain scans support the idea that they have some level of awareness. Patients like that are said to be in "minimally conscious states." Jahi's five-year survival after being declared brain dead has highlighted arguments that the brain death standard is not as objective or as impervious to reasonable dispute as Beecher and many more people since might like. It is a philosophical commitment for us to regard the brain as the central, defining organ of personhood, and therefore brain death as the death of a person, because it both integrates our body's function and enables us to interact with the world around us.

HARVESTING ORGANS

Countries and communities that do not accept brain death have an even harder time procuring scarce organs for transplant than the places that do. To be sure, even in places that have accepted brain death, taking organs from the dead presents ethical challenges that are distinct from taking them from the living. In the United States, deceased persons must either have an advance directive that authorizes taking their viable organs for transplant (including a driver's license or some kind of registry), or else their family must agree. The current system for harvesting organs from the dead requires that those who ask relatives for the organ must be different from those who have taken care of the patient, in order to avoid an actual or perceived conflict of interest. Even that system isn't foolproof. There have been complaints about overly pushy transplant teams.

Many proposals have been offered to increase the supply of organs. They range from less controversial ideas like mounting public education campaigns and making registration as an organ donor easier to more controversial proposals like reimbursement for funeral expenses. Among the most unsettled and consequential questions is whether buying organs from the living or prospectively from the dead is ethical. Rather than foraging for organs, why not buy and sell them on a regulated market? The answer to this question is tied up with the larger one of what we think money should and shouldn't buy, and why?

The most widely used approach worldwide to obtaining transplantable organs from the dead is not simply persuasion or purchase, it's nudging, which we discussed in chapter 3 as an important instrument for furthering public health. Nudging for organs presumes the family's consent unless they or the deceased person has "opted out" of donation. What the nudging approach to organ donation creates is an "opt-out" choice architecture—also known as presumed consent—that aims to increase organ donations, importantly without either forcing or paying people to relinquish their organs. Advocates for "opt out," like the bioethicist Arthur Caplan who has long championed this policy, argue that it increases the contribution rate of lifesaving organs without depriving individuals of the choice to not donate if they (or their families) so choose.

Twenty-five European countries have adopted presumed consent, or opt out, but only a handful have greater donation rates than the United States, which remains "opt in." In some opt-out countries, health care workers still seek the active consent of family members because they think it's unacceptable to take a deceased person's organs if the family objects to the taking. In 2016, Spain—a Catholic country—had the highest rate of deceased organ donors, while the United States trailed behind Spain, Croatia, Portugal, and Belgium. Yet the U.S. rate is still strikingly higher than most other countries that have presumed consent, but not nearly high enough to meet the dire demand.

Many observers credit Spain's program of placing trained transplant coordinators in all of its hospitals for making more of a difference in raising its contribution rate than its opt-out policy. That program is an ethically uncontroversial practice that could raise the donation rates in all countries. There's evidence that major American cities with hospitals that systematically seek donations have significantly higher donor rates than those like the single largest, New York City, with many hospitals that resist organized donation programs.

Major demographic and cultural differences between the United States and European countries make it rash to assume that "opt out" versus "opt in" accounts for overall contribution-rate differences. Here is yet another striking piece of evidence about how we need to face up to values that clash in some social contexts but not others: although most Americans say that they want to be organ donors, it remains an uphill struggle for presumed consent to gain a foothold among a citizenry with so many so deeply resistant to their governments' presuming their agreement to anything they think important. The decision to posthumously donate our organs is truly important, and that is why we would democratically support a system for organ donation that honors our freedom of choice, while nudging us to save lives every day. Most likely, it will take a grassroots movement of concerned, persistent, and persuasive citizens—mounting a captivating campaign that drives home its lifesaving stakes—to move opt-out organ donation forward in the United States.

ALTRUISTIC ORGAN DONATION AND THE MARKET

Americans generally accept the current opt-in policy for organ donations. To the extent that it works, it serves a dual moral mission: it gives life to those who receive the organs and it also gives voice to the virtue of those who donate them, a virtue known as altruism. But something is often overlooked in the zealous defense of an opt-in policy based on altruistic donation. If opt in secures significantly fewer organs than an opt-out policy, we shouldn't want to use it simply to demonstrate altruism, which after all is the motivation to help others. Altruists don't let people needlessly die. And altruism isn't an acceptable alternative to saving more lives. Quite the contrary, the motivation to help others requires us to consider how we can do more to save lives, not only individually but also institutionally. The United States and the world continue to face acute shortages of donated organs. Can we collectively find more effective, ethical ways to minimize needless deaths? It would be a tragic irony if altruism stood in the way of aiding more people. Altruistic motives should support an effective opt-out policy for obtaining organs for transplant.

Faced with profound organ shortages, what else should a democratic society do? Solid organ donation from the living primarily involves kidneys or, in fewer cases, portions of the liver. While the transplant surgeon community in the United States has strongly supported altruistic donation, they have also been struggling with how to alleviate the dire scarcity of lifesaving organs. Just about everything transplant surgeons use to treat their patients is bought and sold, including their own labor and, most strikingly, the donated organs that organ-procurement organizations sell to transplant programs. We have summarized the strong case that is commonly made for relying on altruism—or other nonfinancial motives, such as reciprocity—as a valuable motivation for advance directives to donate after death. No doubt, the United States and other societies could do more to facilitate such other-regarding motivations, perhaps with a program like Spain's that places trained transplant coordinators in all hospitals.

Yet Spain's soft approach, while admirable in principle, might not be as efficient as the market. The ever-widening gap between need-based demand and organ supply calls upon us to consider whether there's an ethically defensible way of paying some donors for organs, or would a payment system be inherently and unavoidably exploitative? Can the sale of organs be regulated to avoid exploitation while maximally ensuring the safety and informed consent of donors? And should it be? The two major, overarching objections to selling human organs are clearly distinguished by political philosopher Michael Sandel. One is broadly based on corruption and the other on unfairness. The corruption objection is the more unconditional: a market in organs, even a regulated market, distorts their meaning by misidentifying them as commodities that we own in much the same way as we own our clothes or cars. Selling organs, the corruption argument goes, degrades and objectifies our personhood by treating us "as a collection of spare parts." (The extreme extension of commodification is selling our entire bodies along with our labor, which is tantamount to freely selling ourselves into slavery.) Under current law and public policy, body parts cannot be sold. In a legal sense we do not own our body or its parts.

But don't we have a right to sell an organ based on our personal freedom? In the spirit of John Stuart Mill's *On Liberty*, might a liberal argue that we have a right to use our bodily parts as we wish, short of using them directly to harm others (or selling ourselves into slavery, which effectively would put an end to our personal freedom)? If our body parts are not commodities in the same sense as our cars, and selling them corrupts their very nature, then the corruption argument against commodification of bodily parts can consistently claim that some significant harm is done, indirectly, to our shared values, relationships, and self-understanding by a society that permits the marketing of human body organs. (Mill himself rejected limiting individual freedom for the sake of protecting against indirect harms.) While the corruption objection to organ sale does not settle the issue, it mounts a reasonable argument for government's role in securing the social value of personhood and noncommodified body parts, by discouraging and maybe even blocking the sale of human organs. A democratic government, on this view, should oppose such corruption even if some people otherwise would freely consent to sell their spare kidneys.

The unfairness objection to the sale of human organs questions whether the transactions would truly be free on the part of the donor. Beyond compensation for incurred costs (which could include forgone income), all payments are deemed unfair. Why? Because markets in human organs unjustly exploit the poor by making them bad offers that, out of desperation, they cannot refuse. When people are desperately poor, bargaining conditions are unfair and markets are not truly voluntary—they "prey upon the poor." We need to note that "preying upon" conveys harm, and for the unfairness objection to be strong enough to override a person's freedom, there must be evidence that serious harm will be done. The unfairness objection cannot consistently be against payment per se—it must be against involuntary or harmful exchanges. In any case, in the absence of extreme poverty and unjust bargaining conditions, as Sandel points out, unfairness withdraws its objection to selling organs, but corruption still opposes their sale as degrading to personhood.

As presented, the general objections from corruption and unfairness both set aside the major aim of obtaining organs for transplant: the chance to save more people's lives. The corruption objection is distinctive in making the case against all market transactions in organs. But it doesn't speak at all to the fact that many organs once donated are then essentially sold by organ procurement organizations that charge "acquisition fees" to transplant centers, which in turn resell them to patients as integral components of transplant service packages. Advocates of a living organ market argue that in the current system everyone makes money except the donor. The National Organ Transplant Act (NOTA)—hastily passed by Congress in 1984 "soon after a former physician announced plans to set up a company to broker human kidneys"—prohibits donors from selling organs for any "valuable consideration." Yet NOTA permits compensation for the costs of organ transplantation, such as their removal, transportation, and implantation. Other costs that seem permissible are for transportation, dependent care, lost wages, insurance for health risks, and life insurance. Compensating donors for these costs is a just, legal, and cost-effective way to increase the supply of organs from living donors. More patients' lives would be saved and extended. And for kidney transplants, savings would include the costs of dialysis.

Even if we suppose that the sale of organs contributes to commodifying some part of personhood, we still need to ask: How does that compare to the chance of saving more lives through a regulated market where, for example, the government offered only informed and healthy donors an in-kind benefit (such as a tax credit or retirement benefit) for donating a kidney to a stranger? The unfairness objection to legally regulated organ sale is more conditional on social context: it diminishes, or even disappears, if those who sell their organs in a regulated market are not poor. That would require a financial background check, by no means a foolproof system.

While the poor are preyed upon today in illegal black markets for organs in poor developing countries, we really don't know who would donate in a highly regulated market in the United States that was designed not only to reward but also to inform and protect donors, and how those donors would fare. We know that by making more healthy organs available and using existing algorithms for distribution, we could greatly benefit low-income individuals in one significant way, since they are overrepresented on the waiting lists for transplants.

ORGANS ABROAD

The Global Observatory on Donation and Transplantation (GODT) reported that over 125,000 solid organs were transplanted in over a hundred countries worldwide in 2015. Unfortunately, this represents only about 10 percent of worldwide requirements for organs. Twenty people on organ waiting lists die every day, having failed to receive an organ. Too often, the fortunate succeed in receiving an organ for reasons other than their immediate medical need. Those reasons might include simply having the social support needed to manage a personal crisis, the financial resources that help them obtain access to prominent physicians, or even celebrity status. In 1995 baseball great Mickey Mantle received a replacement liver just two days after it was requested, raising suspicions about the effectiveness of the system of waiting lists in the United States. Mantle died just two months after his transplant. Some questioned whether at the time of the transplant he was too sick to benefit from such a precious resource and whether that should have been known. Apple founder Steve Jobs, a California resident, was reported to have traveled to Tennessee for a liver transplant. In response to public concerns about fairness in the allocation of livers, the United Network for Organ Sharing (UNOS) put a new policy in place to reduce the unfairness of geographic differences.

In the extreme, solid organs are bought and sold illegally and without any ethical safeguards, known as organ trafficking. In 2012 a married couple arrived in Lahore, Pakistan. Just as the husband was being prepped for transplant, the police burst in and arrested the couple and the well-known surgeons under a 2010 Pakistani law intended to prevent organ trafficking. The law was promulgated by a bioethics institute headed by a female surgeon and ethicist. But enforcement by legal authorities is still a problem. The reality of such organ trafficking is that obtaining organs from living donors, who really are "vendors" in this context, depends on the poverty and vulnerability of the donors. A 2014 UNESCO report estimated that between 5 and 10 percent of transplanted kidneys result from organ trafficking. For cadaveric sources of organs, presumed consent can easily be abused to exploit marginalized, less educated persons and families. They may be reluctant to say they are unwilling to donate out of fear of punitive consequences. These worries don't apply so much to countries with well-regulated systems of organ donation, but ethics cannot be separated from context.

Doesn't blocking the choice of poor individuals to make some needed money by selling a spare kidney only make matters worse for them, wherever they may reside? Evidence suggests that this argument for a "free" market in organs is on shaky empirical ground. Where there is an *unregulated* market for kidneys, reports suggest, people who sell a kidney tend to be worse off in the years following the sale. But, the challenge continues, if the argument against organ sales to the poor is that they cannot freely choose, or they will be exploited, why not also block their market transactions more generally? The answer is because we also consistently value every person's freedom to choose, and most market transactions do not involve their losing something as valuable as a bodily organ. Those transactions that do involve losing something so valuable, such as selling themselves into long and hard labor, justify similar protections by way of regulations (such as maximum work weeks and minimum wage laws) to protect vulnerable individuals against unjust exploitation.

The unfairness objection against organ sales would disappear in a world where background conditions were fair, and no one was so poor and vulnerable as to be able to be unjustly exploited in this way. The corruption objection, by contrast, holds even under ideal conditions of distributive justice. Comparing the two objections for opposing the sale of organs challenges us to consider why some oppose organ sales. Should our opposition persist even in a just and affluent society where income and wealth were fairly distributed? The persistence of poverty and the negative effects of commodification on altruism and other human virtues unite many people in the common cause against the legalized sale of human organs. In an ideal world, we might disagree more!

The case against organ sales remains highly controversial, especially since so many people are understandably desperate for live organ transplants. Some liberals who acknowledge the unfairness and corruption attending organ sales come down in favor of a highly regulated market in organs because of the lives that consequently may be saved. Right now we can only surmise; no one knows whether adding regulated markets to organ donations will increase the overall supply of organs. Social scientists strongly disagree over whether the introduction of some more established markets, such as those in blood donation, have increased or decreased the safe supply of what's also so direly needed.

Consistent with our concern for using evidence-based policy to save more lives, we strongly favor introducing transplant coordinator programs like those that work so effectively in Spain in hospitals where they are now lacking to see how much of a difference such a clearly ethical program can make in organ contribution rates. Depending on how much of a shortfall of organ donations remain, we can also support small and highly regulated demonstration projects on organ sales.

When what's at stake is giving an organ to others who are in dire need, it's not enough to establish whether some people are motivated to give without nudging or payment: some are. We also want to know how many are motivated relative to the need: right now, not nearly enough are, and thousands of primarily middle- and low-income people remain on long wait-lists and die as a consequence. We also need to know how many more or less would be motivated to give if more effective nudging programs were instituted, and if that turns out not to be enough, what would happen if regulated sales were also permitted. Existing evidence strongly supports some nudging programs, like placing transplant coordinators in every hospital. Evidence for regulated sales and their effect on donation and ability to avoid exploitation is sorely insufficient. Not only are the ethical arguments for and against markets highly controversial, so are the empirical findings as to the effect on altruistic giving of introducing markets for some precious goods. Whether a regulated market in kidneys would be neutral, "crowd out," or even "crowd in," altruistic giving is, as legal scholar Julia Mahoney reports, "highly speculative."

Small pilot studies as recommended by the Ethics Committee of the OPTN (Organ Procurement and Transplantation Network) could help discover some probable effects of a federally regulated system of financial incentives and help guide us through what is now a tragic impasse. Depending on the results of these studies, larger randomized controlled trials could be supported or judged not to be worth the time and expense. In the meantime, we should push for all hospitals of significant size to be provided with the modest resources needed to hire well-trained transplant coordinators.

BACK TO FORAGING

Ultimately, the resolution of the natural scarcity of human organs will test our capacity for organizational, scientific, and technological innovation as well as our tolerance for using animals for novel purposes. In 2017, for the first time, geneticists created piglets free of retroviruses with genes that could cause infections in primates. This was a major step toward the possibility of creating a new supply of organs for transplant patients. That precious new supply would come at the price of using another and rather intelligent species as "organ farms"—the same species whose members hundreds of millions of human beings happily eat regularly. For hundreds of millions of others, pork is deliberately abjured, but not out of respect for the animal so much as out of religious belief and injunction that it is unclean.

Is using pigs as an organ source any different from using them as a food source? From many ethical perspectives, there is a difference and it strongly favors use as an organ source. Eating pigs and other animals is a wasteful way of feeding and preserving the planet, and it isn't especially healthy either, while using pig organs may be the best way we have to save lives. It also behooves us to consider how pigs are raised and experimentally treated. If questions of whether and how to use pigs as organ sources seem avoidable now, there likely will be no avoiding them in the future.

Ironically, our ancestors foraged for animal meat to ingest. Now we forage for them to transplant.

Part Three

MORAL
SCIENCE

Seven

HUMAN
EXPERIMENTS

Dying in a London hospital, a baby named Charlie Gard had a rare and severe genetic disorder of the mitochondria, the DNA that is passed down from the mother. Less than a year after he was born in 2017, an international controversy erupted about his treatment. His parents insisted that they should have the chance to try an experimental treatment that had never been used on someone with his condition. Having been informed by Charlie's doctors that death was inevitable, a court ruled that the treatment would only extend his suffering. As the controversy raged, it seemed everybody had an opinion. Even a U.S. president and a pope weighed in. The Charlie Gard case raised many troubling questions, including the ultimate authority of parents to enter their children into a treatment with a remote chance of success.

Using the experimental treatment on Charlie might possibly have brought some new knowledge to light, even if it didn't extend his life. Creating new knowledge is a good thing, undeniably so if it may one day help prevent and treat serious disease. But definitely not so at any price or by any means, such as subjecting someone to added suffering with little or no prospect of benefit and, in the case of children, with no capacity to consent. We stand by this bioethical precept at the same time as we know that for every new breakthrough of knowledge in scientific experimentation on human beings, there has to be a first user.

Under what conditions is it ethical to do a potentially socially important experiment on a human being? There's no better example of the tensions that bioethicists study than those that pervade experimental medicine. Some laboratory animals model human diseases remarkably well, but in the final analysis a rodent is not a human being. There are also, appropriately, many ethical constraints on animals in research. Computer scientists are working on mathematical models of disease processes that might someday minimize and even replace lab animals, providing far greater confidence about the potential effects on human patients. But that day is some years away.

WHAT PRICE KNOWLEDGE?

The ethics of human experiments is far from a new topic. The finest of motives can drive the desire to experiment, as medical doctors have always wanted to improve their understanding of illness in order to better their medical practice. The very idea that doctors "practice" medicine captures the imperfections of medical care. Like in other professions, in medicine there is always more to learn. At the same time, doctors have also puzzled about the ethical limits of experimenting on their patients. The writings often attributed to the ancient medical cult of Hippocrates include passages that still express the dilemma fairly well. When the patient's condition is grave, ancient physicians were advised to "be bold," yet they were also told to "first, do no harm." In a way, those constraints still apply to the ethical framework of modern medicine. As in so much of human life, the fundamental moral challenges we face have changed less than we often think and are more complex than we or our simple proverbs often admit.

For millennia, what happened between doctors and patients was typically known only to them, and the truth about the patient's condition was often known only to the doctor. This meant that doctors had almost unlimited discretion in deciding how to treat their patients. In recent decades, the formerly closed consulting room has been opened up to highly skilled nurses, pharmacists, social workers, medical technologists, students, and insurance companies, not to mention the new profession of hospital ethicist. Before all of those new faces showed up at the bedside in the twentieth century, an even more monumental change occurred in doctor-patient relations in the nineteenth century, when the art of medicine gradually became more science based.

In the 1800s, the renowned Harvard philosopher and psychologist William James followed the path of many of his fellow American medical students to advance his education. Like them, he journeyed to Germany, where he received actual exposure to patients, something the lecture-based American medical schools didn't offer. He also learned about the new physiological psychology being done in places like Berlin, which helped him become a forerunner of modern brain science. Another American named Henry Wellcome, confident that drug research could be based on science rather than snake oil, went to London where he founded one of the world's great drug companies. Though pills had been produced by others, his manufacture and marketing innovations of the "tabloid" pill helped create the modern pharmaceutical industry.

Developments like these were based on experiments and they made more experimental science possible. They also raised awareness of the ethical issues inherent in attempts to advance medical science. Both Americans and Europeans wrote codes of ethics. In 1900 the American Army doctor Walter Reed wrote what we would today call a consent form for people who agreed to be bitten by mosquitoes as part of his yellow fever experiments in Cuba—the first time in history that a medical experiment required written, signed consent. That same year Prussia enacted ethics rules following a scandal about syphilis experiments. The pace picked up in the first decades of the twentieth century. In 1917 a Polish physician published a book called *Medical Ethics* in which he strongly criticized his colleagues for being reckless with their patients. Similar statements, codes, and regulations appeared elsewhere in Europe and in the United States.

Following newspaper reports about unethical tuberculosis experiments, Germany in 1931 established its own guidelines that were in many ways the strictest and most sophisticated in the world. But within two years, Hitler took power and gradually many of the laws of democratic Germany fell by the wayside. With the outbreak of World War II, Hitler's Germany initiated brutal experiments in concentration camps, many intended to solve medical problems that were hampering the Nazi war effort. Victims were frozen to death to learn how to treat hypothermia, suffocated in low-pressure chambers, poisoned by being forced to drink only seawater, and forced to undergo experimental tissue transplant surgery, among other horrors. The fog of war provided a convenient cover. The fact that medical doctors were the perpetrators compounded the shock when the Nazis' crimes were brought to light, a fact made even more troubling considering that German medicine was the most advanced in the world, with what were once the highest ethical standards of the time.

THE DOCTORS' TRIAL

From late 1946 to mid-1947, twenty-three Nazi doctors and bureaucrats were tried in an United States–led international tribunal in Nuremberg, Germany. The fact that this was the first trial after that of the surviving political and military leaders was telling. Emphasizing the outrages of heinous medical experiments, the chief lawyer for the prosecution, General Telford Taylor, asserted in his opening statement to the court that "this is no mere murder trial." But what might have been considered an open-and-shut case based on the extensive evidence turned into a more complicated process as the Nazis' defense lawyers made their arguments. Over weeks of testimony, they produced examples of human experiments conducted by the Allied countries and others that they claimed were no less questionable than those in the camps. One of those cases was described in a 1945 *Life* magazine photo-essay. It described a White House–sponsored malaria experiment with hundreds of prisoners in the Stateville Penitentiary near Joliet, Illinois. The experiment's purpose was to find a better treatment for malaria before the United States and its allies faced the grim prospect of invading the home islands of Japan, an invasion that never took place because Japan sued for peace after the nuclear devastation of Hiroshima and Nagasaki.

In the end, the judges didn't find the defense arguments persuasive. Some of the experiments cited by the Nazi doctors' lawyers were in the open medical literature, while the Nazis kept their experiments as secret as they could, and for contemptible reasons. In the camps, death was the expected result, even intended in many cases. When the victims didn't die, they were often killed, sometimes so that they couldn't bear witness. And unlike the Nazi experiments, the malaria experiment was not only quite public (the *Life* magazine article about the experiment turned out to be a propaganda coup for the government and for the prison), it qualified as voluntary under the conventions of the day and was overseen by qualified medical doctors. Years later, the ability of even regular prisoners to "volunteer" for experiments would be debated and ultimately found to be acceptable only under very strict and specific conditions.

Finally, the court returned to the real issue in the case, that at least some of the defendants were responsible for cruel deaths and injuries. Seven of them were sentenced to hang for their crimes. The judges also noted that the rules for doing human experiments needed to be clarified. As part of their judgment in the case, they included a ten-point set of ethical rules that have come to be known as the Nuremberg Code. The first line of the code states that "the voluntary consent of the human subject is absolutely essential." Other elements of the code include the requirement that the experiment should be important, that it should be based on previous knowledge such as from animal experiments, and that the subjects must be free to withdraw from the experiment at any time.

The Doctors' Trial, as it has come to be known, was only moderately covered in U.S. newspapers as it unfolded. But, on the whole, many Americans and many in Europe were more than ready to move on from two catastrophic world wars. The lessons of the Nazi period were by no means all easy to learn at first. In the case of American doctors, the concentration camp experiments were hard to fathom and the Nuremberg Code seemed largely unnecessary. Jay Katz recalled the reactions of his medical school professors: they thought, he said, that it was a good ethics code for barbarians but irrelevant to legitimate medical science.

Now we know that the trial did have one immediate effect on American medical ethics. While the defense lawyers were making their case, wishing to insulate U.S. medicine from any association with the Nazi doctors, the American Medical Association's expert witness, Dr. Andrew Ivy, arranged for an Illinois governor's committee to adopt a code of ethics that the AMA had published in small print in the December 1946 issue of their journal. A few months later, Ivy returned to Germany to affirm on the witness stand that Americans did have such a code, though he did not mention that it had just been introduced or that he was its author.

TWENTY-TWO CASES

Henry Beecher, who in the late 1960s led the Harvard committee that established the brain death standard, was still a young anesthesiologist after his World War II service. The U.S. Army asked him to review some information from the Buchenwald concentration camp. Beecher responded in a report that was then classified:

Near the building used as a hospital was a pathological laboratory. I saw specimens of pulmonary tuberculosis, carcinoma of the lung and tattooed [*sic*] skin. These were put up in regular museum jars, and were unusual in no way. It was evident, however, from the attention they excited, that they were looked upon by non-medical visitors as illustrations of the depravity of the German doctors . . . In this building, however, it seems clear that ruthless experiments on live human beings were carried on. Dr. Ding, a well-known German clinician, is said to have tested a typhus vaccine here on human beings, by inoculating them with a vaccine and injecting them with a live virulent culture later. The experiment was unsuccessful. One report was that 900 were inoculated and 700 died. Whatever the numbers, there appears no question about the basic facts.

Over the next years, Beecher's interest in the ethics of human experiments intensified. He was not convinced that the concentration camp experiments were entirely unique. In the early 1960s, he warned in general terms that attitudes about the use of human subjects were too casual, perhaps sensing that a crisis in public awareness of the issue was sure to erupt at some point. Apparently deciding that a more specific statement had to be made, with case examples, he submitted a paper to the *Journal of the American Medical Association* that listed fifty unethical experiments. The journal politely turned him down. Then he approached the editor of the *New England Journal of Medicine*. Over objections from the editorial board, the *NEJM* editor accepted the paper with a pared-down list of twenty-two examples of what he considered to be unethical human experiments in the published medical literature, but without specific references. Beecher and the editor agreed that naming those who had done the experiments would be a distraction from the important point about ethics and that the authors of those papers might even be subject to legal action.

Beecher's paper stunned the medical world. It was one thing to prosecute Nazis for unethical experiments, but quite another thing for a distinguished member of the medical establishment to call out his colleagues. And some of the cases were easily recognizable even though their investigators were not identified. One of them was a study that involved exposing debilitated elderly patients to live cancer cells. The Brooklyn Jewish Chronic Disease Hospital case was led by a well-known doctor from Manhattan's famous Memorial Sloan Kettering Cancer Center, Chester Southam, who wondered how the immune systems of compromised people would respond to foreign cancer cells. Neither the patients nor their families were told the real nature of the study. New York State sanctioned two of the doctors, an unheard-of punishment in those days of deference to physicians. But the sanction was still pretty weak—just probation. And Dr. Southam went on to be the president of a major cancer research organization several years later.

The Brooklyn Jewish Chronic Disease Hospital case, which broke in 1964, illustrated the problem of limits to acquiring new knowledge. Even if the elderly patients experienced no physical harm, they were wronged by being made part of an experiment without consent. A director of the hospital pleaded in court for disclosure of the medical records saying that "the patients . . . were used as guinea pigs." For the rest of his life, Dr. Southam argued that the study was legitimate, but it's undeniable that the elderly patients' bodies were being used *merely* as physiological laboratories. That's what it means to be used as a guinea pig. They had neither consented to this treatment nor did they have anything to gain from it. Many both inside and outside of medicine were beginning to think that respect for human subjects of medical experiments had to be taken more seriously. The Brooklyn episode was a clear case of an unethical medical experiment. But another case on Beecher's list still arouses heated debate.

WILLOWBROOK AND TUSKEGEE

In the late 1950s a distinguished New York University hepatitis researcher named Saul Krugman began clinical studies at the Willowbrook State School on New York's Staten Island. The school, home to thousands of children with intellectual and physical disabilities, was plagued by outbreaks of infectious hepatitis, especially as rapidly growing demand for its services led to severe overcrowding and as living conditions deteriorated. With funding from the U.S. armed forces, Krugman hoped to find a way to prevent hepatitis A, which normally causes short-term illness but can lead to death. He deliberately exposed some children to the virus by giving them "milk shakes" containing fecal material from infected children. As conditions in the school were disclosed by the New York City media, Krugman's experiments were also criticized by those who claimed that parents were pressured to agree to allow their children into the experiments in order to be assured of a place at the school.

In his 1966 exposé Beecher summarized Krugman's studies at Willowbrook as one of the twenty-two unethical human experiments. Krugman argued that his experiment was justified partly because the children would likely have gotten hepatitis anyway, that they would be immunized, and that the parents consented. To the end of his life, Krugman contended that the experiments were ethical, and even today he continues to have defenders. In a way, Krugman was an especially formidable opponent of Beecher. Like Beecher, Krugman was an important academic who had made basic contributions to his field (in Krugman's case distinguishing between hepatitis A and B). But the Willowbrook episode also drew attention to a broader question, equally relevant to the ethics of human experiments: What is the context in which human experiments are done? The institutional environment at the school was deplorable, including physical and sexual abuse of the children by staff. Under such conditions, conducting ethical experiments becomes impossible. No matter how much anyone might want to take advantage of an opportunity to gain knowledge that can prevent human suffering, some settings are ethically unacceptable.

There is no more telling example of exploiting the corrupt setting for human experimentation in the history of bioethics in the United States than the Tuskegee syphilis study. The Tuskegee experiments were not a secret within the Public Health Service or the medical research community. They lasted four decades, from 1932 through 1972, and directly involved 600 African American sharecroppers, 399 of whom had previously contracted syphilis but were never told by the "professional" medical researchers, working for the U.S. government, that they had the disease. Nor were they ever treated with penicillin long after it was known to be a proven treatment. All were manipulated into cooperation by being told that they needed to be periodically examined—and sometimes have spinal taps—because they had "bad blood." They were not respected as persons, let alone treated, even paternalistically, as patients, to say the least. Instead, as the *New York Times* reported on July 26, 1972, "human beings . . . were induced to serve as guinea pigs." Nearly six years had passed since a sexually transmissible disease investigator named Peter Buxton first complained about the study to the Centers for Disease Control. Finally, he decided to go to the press. In the wake of the public revelations, a blue-ribbon panel was formed. It declared the experiments unethical from their inception and recommended their immediate termination and the commencement of any treatment needed by the survivors.

The term "bombshell" might be overused, but that was the way the Tuskegee revelations hit the country. Coming on the heels of the African American civil rights movement, the syphilis study confirmed that systemic racism affected even the medical establishment and had done so since notorious experiments on black slaves. Historians have shown that pre–Civil War Southern medical schools exploited the presence of enslaved persons for experimentation. Some Northern medical schools, including our own, educated students from the South who returned to practice medicine on enslaved people and who circulated pro-slavery ideas. The case of a famous Southern gynecologist, J. Marion Sims, has been especially heinous. Before the Civil War, Sims developed an improved speculum for vaginal examinations, which were done rarely and reluctantly, and pioneered a surgical treatment for a painful condition in which the bladder and uterus are torn following childbirth. However, his first patients were relatively available black enslaved individuals who were volunteered by their owners, and the procedures were done without anesthesia on the theory that blacks felt less pain than whites. Sims also conducted experimental surgeries with black children. In 2018, 124 years after it was erected, a statue of Sims was removed from New York's Central Park.

Proverbially speaking, history casts long shadows. It wasn't until

1974 that two decades of experiments at the mostly black Holmes-burg Prison in Philadelphia ended. By the early 1970s, medical research involving fetuses and genetic manipulation, as well as African Americans, prisoners, mental patients, and other vulnerable populations, was cause for bipartisan concern. Since the late 1960s, several members of Congress had called for some kind of national commission to review America's human experiments practices. The Tuskegee panel called for creating a national board to regulate all federally supported research with human subjects. While Congress did not create a national regulatory board, Democrats and Republicans joined together to pass legislation, signed by President Nixon only months before his resignation in 1974, creating America's first nationwide bioethics commission, the National Commission for the Protection of Human Subjects of Biomedical and Behavioral Research, as we mentioned in chapter 2. In operation from 1974 to 1978, the commission produced a number of influential reports and recommendations that became federal regulations, especially concerning vulnerable populations like children and prisoners.

The resulting federal "common rule" required prior review of a proposed experiment by an institutional review board (IRB)—a better name would be "research ethics board," the term used in much of the world—and informed consent by the research volunteers. (The National Institutes of Health and some hospitals had already employed IRBs for some time, so the practice wasn't entirely new.) In the words of the physician Jerome Groopman, himself a prominent cancer and HIV researcher, "we need such guardrails to protect patients not only from extreme risks from experimental therapies to the quality and longevity of their lives but also from distorted judgment resulting from a doctor's mixed emotions of compassion and ambition." Revelations about experiments conducted before the creation of the IRB system demonstrate how much it is needed, and problems with experiments conducted even after its creation demonstrate that it's far from foolproof.

THE HUMAN RADIATION EXPERIMENTS

In 1994 the *Albuquerque Tribune*'s Eileen Welsome won the Pulitzer Prize for documenting long-rumored injections of hospitalized patients with plutonium during and immediately after World War II. Their purpose: to determine how to detect plutonium in the human body, including by examining excreta. The decision to expose sick patients was the path of least resistance for the directors of the project to build the atomic bomb, since their laboratory workers were also being exposed to this new metal that is far more radioactive than uranium. Strange as it may seem, this was a worker safety experiment. Because the plutonium experiment was conducted by the federal government with eighteen vulnerable American citizens and covered up for decades, alarmed members of his administration brought it to President Bill Clinton. Other experiments involving ionizing radiation were also known to have taken place since the war years and up through the early 1970s. President Clinton appointed a commission under the leadership of bioethicist Ruth Faden.* The commission's charge was both to find the facts and to determine whether such things could happen under the current regulations and ethical standards.

Working exhaustively for eighteen months, and with presidential authority to request rapid release of classified materials, the advisory committee found a dizzying array of government-sponsored radiation experiments. Not only plutonium, but also uranium, polonium, radioisotopes, and total body irradiation were objects of study. The affected populations and intentional human subjects included prisoners, military personnel, Native Americans, Spanish Americans, children, and cancer patients. In some cases, the advisory committee recommended compensation for the victims or their survivors, ranging from an official apology to financial compensation, depending on

---

* Jonathan was a staff member of the Advisory Committee for Human Radiation Experiments in 1994–1995.

the severity of the ethical offense. None of the plutonium injection patients died of the radiation exposure, but their bodies were used as laboratories without their consent, justifying compensation. The Navajo who worked in the uranium mines and mills, many of whom died prematurely of lung cancer, were not warned of the radiation risks for many years. Not even inexpensive measures were employed to reduce their risks. The miners were entitled to financial compensation. The commission found that strengthened research protections like those in the Belmont Report would not be a guarantee of ethical conduct. They recommended that the government thoroughly examine the processes and the real outcomes of the research protection system.

One aspect of the radiation experiments sets them apart: they took place under the banner of U.S. national security. Had the lawyers for the Nazi doctors known about the plutonium injections, they would surely have added them to their list of defense exhibits, though judges would not have been fooled by the false analogy with a systematic and racist death industry. Yet the fact remains that these and many other experiments on radiation, as well as in other domains like chemical weapons, were rationalized by national security concerns and were covered up to prevent embarrassment to the government. National security claims continue to play a poorly understood role in rationalizing unethical human experiments. Often this can be seen most clearly in the rearview mirror.

GUATEMALA

We were both involved in a case that brought home for us the way that history lives on in the present day, even over what we thought were settled cases in bioethics. While we were working in our respective roles on President Barack Obama's bioethics commission, historian Susan Reverby reported a stunning discovery, one that stimulated a commission report. Reverby was following up her previous research on the Tuskegee syphilis study when she found documents about

U.S. Public Health Service experiments in Guatemala from 1946 to 1948. These experiments were conducted in cooperation with Guatemalan officials, and they exposed prisoners, sex workers, mental patients, soldiers, and in at least one case even a child to sexually transmissible diseases. One of the American doctors involved would go on to be part of the Tuskegee syphilis study.

One purpose of the Guatemala experiments was to determine whether penicillin and other drugs would prevent infection from syphilis, gonorrhea, or chancroid. At that time, paid sex was legal in Guatemala. The experiments deliberately exposed sex workers to gonorrhea or syphilis, and then they had unprotected sex with prisoners. But the doctors determined that there were too few infections for the study, so they decided to also use mental hospital patients, soldiers, and prisoners, exposing them by injection and by exposing the penis to the infectious material. Large numbers of subjects were involved, ultimately almost fifteen hundred. Finally, the project encountered so many problems, like failures in transmission rates, that whatever results it might have produced became irrelevant as the benefits of penicillin were becoming obvious anywhere that doctors had access to it.

The shock that was registered in both the United States and Guatemala when these experiments were discovered in 2010 can be explained at many levels. The president's commission could not find any evidence of consent on the part of the people whose bodies were used without concern about the long-term health consequences for them if the antibiotic didn't work. Poor, mentally ill, institutionalized, and often from native populations, these individuals were among the most vulnerable people in the world. They were, as in so many other cases, used merely as human laboratories with no modicum of respect for them as persons. Remarkably, a similar experiment at an Indiana prison several years before, one not involving sex workers, did require that the prisoners be volunteers, but there was no such requirement in Guatemala.

Were the people responsible for the Guatemala study aware that they were in violation of the ethics of the day? In fact, the commission didn't need to worry about projecting twenty-first-century ethics on a twentieth-century experiment. As the commission pored over the documents from the experiments, they found both internal memos and newspaper articles that made it clear that the Public Health Service officials and doctors responsible for the experiments knew full well that they were playing fast and loose with the ethics, and that the way the experiments were done would not have been acceptable in the United States. They had no interest in making the experiments known for fear of the public reaction. A careless attitude and a de facto cover-up were evident at the highest levels of the U.S. Public Health Service.

Yet the problems being addressed were real threats to public health as sexually transmissible diseases (STDs) were rampant both in the civilian world and in the military. STDs were a special problem for the U.S. Navy in the Pacific during World War II, when the National Research Council expected millions of lost man-days per year, the equivalent of two armored divisions and ten aircraft carriers a year. Here again, national security was likely a motivating rationale for the experiments, especially in an era when the prospects for conflict with the Soviet Union, hard on the heels of World War II, could not be ruled out. Six decades later, Guatemala became the first occasion for a U.S. president to issue a formal apology to the president of a sovereign nation for using their people in an unethical and reprehensible experiment.

ERODING PUBLIC TRUST

Many of the National Commission's recommendations about protecting people in research were made part of federal regulations, including special requirements for vulnerable populations like children and prisoners. From the early 1980s to the late 1990s, many had a sense that the worst excesses of unethical human experiments were behind us, that the system of informed consent and ethics review boards had helped turn a corner. Then came a crushing reminder that as science embodies our aspirations it may also come at an unacceptable cost, in something far more morally weighty than money. Since the 1970s, many research scientists and clinicians hoped that a new kind of medical treatment would be made possible by the ability to recombine genes in a patient's cells. With the prospect of gene therapy, their abstract hopes for this new approach to often untreatable diseases began to materialize. More concrete options emerged as their understanding of the human genome grew and lab techniques became more precise. By the late 1990s, the ground seemed ripe for experiments that could find their way into clinical use.

One genetic disorder with tragic consequences for most affected children attracted the attention of scientists and physicians at the University of Pennsylvania as a candidate for gene therapy. A liver disease called OTC deficiency hampers the ability to metabolize ammonia. Although babies with OTC deficiency rarely survive infancy, a young man named Jesse Gelsinger was less seriously affected. In 1999 he volunteered to try a gene therapy in the hopes that the knowledge gained might help the babies. He was injected with a virus designed to carry what was thought to be a treatment to correct the DNA in his liver. Instead he suffered a massive response of his immune system that resulted in his death several days later. The FDA found that measurements of Jesse's liver should have precluded him from the study and that bad reactions from previous subjects and deaths of monkeys should have been disclosed. The tragedy of his death was compounded by public outrage that one of the investigators and the university had a financial stake in the experimental treatment.

Less than two years after Jesse Gelsinger died, a healthy volunteer for an experiment at Johns Hopkins University also lost her life, in 2001. Ellen Roche was a twenty-four-year-old technician at Hopkins' asthma center who agreed to inhale a drug that induces mild asthma as part of a study of natural defenses in healthy people. Instead of the expected small reaction, Roche's lungs began to fail. She died after weeks in the intensive care unit. After her death, experts who were not part of the study concluded that the drug, hexamethonium, was known to be dangerous. They charged that the experimenters did sloppy research on the drug, which was no longer approved by the FDA (and was never approved for inhalation) and found fault with the informed consent form.

The effects of these cases on science were enormous. Research on fifteen thousand human subjects at Hopkins was suspended after the Roche case. Gelsinger's death created a crisis in gene therapy research. It also brought new scrutiny to the role of money in modern medical research. Big medical breakthroughs typically trace their origins back to scientific labs that are university and government funded where basic, preclinical research hypotheses are rigorously tested. This early-stage research, whose results may be patentable, is far less often funded by private industry because the profit-making proposition is long term and speculative. The bipartisan 1980 Bayh-Dole Act was a key incentive for this system, which has been very productive for medical research. By allowing universities, small businesses, and nonprofit organizations to own, patent, and license their federally funded inventions, the law encouraged the downstream development and commercialization of discoveries that might otherwise sit on the shelf.

If preclinical testing suggests that a new treatment may work safely on people, three phases of clinical trials generally need to be undertaken with human participants. The early testing focuses on safety and dosage, and then later on efficacy and side effects for larger numbers of patients. The final preapproval studies—the Phase III trials—typically involve gathering data from hundreds if not thousands of people. Clinical trials are extremely expensive and dependent upon significant private or public funding. Private industry is more likely to fund clinical trials than upstream research and to do so in exchange for the legal rights to market the treatment if proven safe, efficacious, and better than the current standard (and approved by the FDA). The patent holders also usually share in the downstream profits, so the potential exists all along the way for interested parties—many with financial conflicts of interest—to underestimate the importance of ethical standards.

The ethical requirements for clinical research center around obtaining safety and efficacy approvals and the informed consent of human subjects. Regardless of how motivated academic researchers are by the public good they can do with their next clinical breakthrough, they are rightly bound by rigorous regulatory requirements that assure safety, efficacy, and informed consent. It would be both dangerous and foolish to treat these controls as meddlesome bureaucratic barriers rather than as important means of earning public support. Regulatory requirements and institutional controls help to mitigate conflicts of interest, even if the ethical tensions inherent in commercializing biomedical research cannot be completely eliminated. Since the 1990s, much tighter institutional controls have been put in place with this essential purpose of mitigating conflicts of interest and their appearance in medical research.

Some argue that the era of low-hanging fruit in medical science has passed, that breakthroughs like the polio vaccines were largely matters of trial and error and depended on the ability to involve large numbers of people at relatively low cost. Medical breakthroughs typically take a lot of time, the costs of research have increased, and the short-term financial incentives to shortcut ethical standards are undeniable. Despite these formidable hurdles to ethically translating research into patient care, the early twenty-first century has already been judged one of the most productive periods in recent history for new drugs, innovative biomedical devices, and cancer breakthroughs. And precisely because of the formidable hurdles, never has there been a greater need for medical science, economics, and ethics to join forces in enabling affordable life-enhancing and lifesaving progress.

The Gelsinger and Roche deaths undermined confidence at the close of the twentieth century that milestones like the Nuremberg Code and the Belmont Report had turned the corner on ethical issues in human experiments. A significant part of the problem was that the institutional complexities along with the financial costs of engaging

in biomedical research were rapidly changing and the institutionalized ethics processes hadn't caught up. If anything, those challenges
are even greater now. Translations of very complex theories in fields
like genetics into disease treatments involve many highly trained and
specialized people using sophisticated equipment. This raises costs
while multiplying the challenges of ensuring that everyone understands and embraces their ethical obligations. Public demands for
speedy and less regulated progress are also far greater, as we discussed
in chapter 6 in the case of misnamed "right-to-try" laws for access
to new experimental drugs. A common denominator in all of these
stories is that our scientific reach must not be allowed to exceed our
moral grasp.

EARNING PUBLIC TRUST

In an open society, the public's trust in science as an ethical enterprise is crucial. "Letting science rip" at the price of needlessly losing
lives is not an acceptable option. Jesse Gelsinger's death discouraged
human experiments in gene therapy for quite a few years. Yet little more than a decade later, a breakthrough in the application of
modern genetics saved the lives of terminally ill cancer patients who
had been unresponsive to every traditional therapy. In 2011 the *New
England Journal of Medicine* published headline-grabbing results of
successful immunotherapy research led by Carl June (at the University of Pennsylvania) that drew upon decades of worldwide research,
including his own earlier HIV studies. June used modified HIV to
alter the DNA of each patient's T cells, a kind of white blood cell
involved in the immune system, creating "chimeras" that both search
out and destroy cancer cells. Once these "chimeric anitigen receptor
cells," or CAR-T cells, kill the patient's cancer cells, they remain on
surveillance, ready to kill any new cancer cells.

A clinical trial at the Children's Hospital of Philadelphia (CHOP)
with children who had acute lymphoblastic leukemia had a 90 percent success rate. The first patient in that trial, six-year-old Emily

Whitehead, experienced a violent immune-system reaction. It wasn't at all obvious at the time, but it turns out that Emily was experiencing a "cytokine storm," which would have killed her were it not for her doctors' decision to try an additional drug, Tocilizumab, that had never before been used in this kind of situation. Coincidentally, June knew about this drug because it had worked for his daughter's arthritis against the same target. The team would soon learn that many patients experience this violent reaction, so the use of this drug turned out to be essential to the treatment's success.* By conservative estimates, FDA-approved CAR-T therapies are poised to benefit tens of thousands.

Emily and others like her are among the minority of young leukemia patients who had not benefited from other advances in the treatment of this disease since the 1960s. In the 1960s, when we were in high school, 90 percent of children with leukemia died. Since then, those numbers have been reversed, and 90 percent survive. Gene therapy could mean that the death rate will be brought to zero, saving the lives of around six hundred children each year in the United States alone. The once experimental treatment became approved therapy, marketed as Kymriah by the multinational drug company Novartis. It is startlingly expensive (an important issue to which we return). Now that it, too, is no longer experimental, insurers will need to consider covering it as they do bone marrow transplants, which are similarly expensive. As the FDA reasoned, it clearly satisfies an "unmet need" for a previously "devastating and deadly" disease.

To understand both the promise and the challenge of ethical human experimentation, it's important to consider what might have happened had Emily's doctors not been able to administer Tocilizumab quickly enough to her. It was, after all, a time-sensitive judg-

---

* As we write this, Emily is now a vibrant, cancer-free twelve-year old; hundreds of other patients are in remission (receiving periodic blood infusions to maintain their immune systems); and the FDA gave its first approvals ever to gene therapies for cancer, but by no means its last ones.

ment call. As June put it, "if the first patient dies on a protocol and nobody's been cured, you're over." Like many highly motivated research scientists and dedicated doctors, he worries that there is not "enough leeway for side effects when you have a potentially curative therapy." The correlative concern, as illustrated by the Charlie Gard case, is that desperate individuals must be protected from entering themselves or their children into overly risky experiments with too little demonstrated upside potential and too great a risk of seriously negative side effects—death after prolonged suffering from an unproven treatment being the ultimate negative side effect. The FDA approval of CAR-T therapies in 2017 exemplifies both just how much it takes and how much can be gained by forging an ethical pathway to advancing lifesaving knowledge.

The development of CAR-T therapy also exemplifies the high costs that accompany many breakthrough treatments in twenty-first-century medicine. It's a case study, yet to be fully written, in just how much talent, team effort, time, and money it takes, and also in just how much can be gained by forging an ethical pathway to advancing lifesaving knowledge. When it comes to developing new knowledge about serious diseases, we cannot escape the question: What costs are and are not justified?

We begin with what's more valuable than money: an ethical human experiment obtains informed consent from participants (or from legal guardians for those who cannot consent), and it must not impose disproportionate risks (relative to anticipated benefits) on anyone. Still controversial is what counts as a disproportionate risk in a therapeutically promising but unproven experiment for terminally ill patients who have exhausted all proven therapies. Because pathbreaking biomedical science is extremely costly, many people must invest in it for progress to be possible. They also typically stand to gain from its success. Ethical professionals conducting human experiments govern themselves by rules set by nonpartisan governmental agencies like the FDA, even when some rules are not precisely to their own liking. Drug companies also need to step up to the plate.

International ethical codes call for "benefit sharing." In that spirit, following a successful clinical trial on life-threatening or serious diseases, the participants need to be assured that they will continue to receive the product if they and their doctors think it has helped them. The company owes posttrial access to the people who agreed to be a part of the study until they can be transitioned to another way of acquiring the product.

The perspective of deliberative democracy calls for public as well as expert input into rule making about human experiments. Why? Because it increases the likelihood that ethics and science will progress together over time. Deliberation can improve the quality of decision making at the same time as it demonstrates respect for the many stakeholders in bioethical decisions. When science proudly partners with ethics—bringing out into the open all that is at stake in moving forward with pathbreaking science for the public good—democracies have the greatest chance of not erring either on the side of too much caution or too little in experiments to find cures for deadly diseases. The more medical science progresses by both being informed by ethics and informing ethics, the clearer it will become that both kinds of errors—too much precaution or too little—can be similarly deadly.

Any prospect of death has a way of commanding human attention. When the prospect involves unknown probabilities, multiple motivated enemies, and millions of unprotected children as possible targets, the question of what our society should do to protect them takes on a sense of urgency. When the only known means of protection is a vaccine that has yet to be tested for its safety or efficacy on children, then urgency comes coupled with controversy. In 2012 Secretary of Health and Human Services Kathleen Sebelius asked President Obama's bioethics commission (on which, as mentioned, we both served) to deliver "rational, independent, evidence-based advice [to] . . . develop a pathway to figure out how to keep our children safe and secure in the event that something occurs"—the "something" being an anthrax attack against the United States. The issue was not theoretical. Such an attack had already occurred a few weeks after 9/11 through envelopes containing anthrax spores, resulting in the deaths of five people and infections in seventeen more. All of the victims were adults, but what if they had included children? While a safe adult anthrax vaccine existed, there is no simple, surefire way to translate safe dosages for adults to children.

Two opposing sides lined up on this issue of the ethics of human experimentation. The national security establishment pressed to move ahead rapidly in testing the anthrax vaccine in children. Otherwise, in the event of an anthrax attack, children would die. Many advocates for children countered that with too little known about the test's safety, the tested children would be subject to serious risks of adverse reactions without corresponding benefits. No child (or adult, for that matter) should be used as a guinea pig.

In contrast to gene therapy, these experiments have no direct prospect of benefit to their participants. In the anthrax-testing case, the participants would be children who are tested before any attack threatens them (or is reliably predicted to do so). By widely accepted and federally instituted standards, experiments with no direct benefit to vulnerable participants should generally proceed only when there is minimal risk, roughly meaning a risk no greater than what most people reasonably and routinely take in their daily lives. Two opposing questions are inescapable: How does a humane society justify more than minimal risk when there is no proportionate benefit for the individual, especially when those individuals are children? And how does a humane society justify leaving all children unprotected in the event of a deadly future attack when the risk of testing anthrax vaccine on a few children is far from life-threatening? Whenever possible, we want to protect many children from a deadly biological attack while also protecting a few from bearing disproportionate risks for the sake of protecting the many.

After extensive and open public deliberations, informed by both scientific evidence and ethical reasoning, the bioethics commission recommended an ethical way of proceeding that no major side had proposed: first test the vaccine, which is known to be safe in adults, in the youngest adults, then provided there's a finding of safety, do so in the oldest minors, and then the next to the oldest, and so on. Such progressive age de-escalation is designed so that it presents no exceptional ethical challenge to testing the vaccine in children because at no stage will it be any more than minimal risk for those at each stage. When science partners with ethics in painstaking public deliberations, new ways are found to protect the public, but not at the expense of unjustifiable harm to innocent people.

Eight

REPRODUCTIVE
TECHNOLOGIES

Nothing is more important to a new parent than a healthy baby. But that's not all. Besides noticing the more obvious features in the minutes after birth, many of us find ourselves counting the fingers and toes, thus audibly or mentally pronouncing the baby "perfect." What counts as perfection, however, is far more complicated than it might first appear. Even for those of us who are not natural gamblers, the reproductive process is essentially a lottery, and one in which we fully expect to love the outcome no matter what it is. Perhaps remarkably, we really do. We intensely love our children for who they are, for all their "perfect imperfections," and not for some predetermined plan of who they will be. As the weeks, months, and years roll on, parental love is often stressed, but it's nearly always unconditional. It begins with a reproductive lottery.

WHAT IS A PARENT?

New reproductive technologies, though, are challenging the nature of that lottery. For those who want no part of reproduction, modern birth control measures have made it easier and safer to avoid being part of the reproductive lottery at all. For those who think they should wait for a time to conceive when they feel better prepared to raise children, modern birth control also offers an invaluable freedom. If an individual or couple does want to play the lottery but for a wide range of reasons is unable to do so, conception through the union of egg and sperm can, as the last decades have come to reveal, be accomplished in a laboratory.

Since 1978, millions of babies have been produced through in vitro fertilization (IVF). Though techniques for artificial insemination to produce "turkey-baster babies" have been around since time immemorial, they can't compete with IVF for efficiency and they don't work at all if the parents suffer from certain conditions. No sooner had Louise Brown been born near Manchester, England, in 1978 than some religious leaders worried about a future of scientifically spawned "Frankenbabies." According to Brown's autobiography, amid the largely congratulatory messages, her parents also received hate mail. Much ignorant speculation abounded about her ultimate characteristics, her personal future, and her own ability to have children. That last question was settled when Brown gave birth to her first child, produced the old-fashioned way.

Whatever controversy surrounded IVF, a child custody case that became a cause célèbre less than a decade after Louise Brown's birth was a glaring reminder that ideas about who counted as a parent were being challenged in ways that didn't necessarily involve fancy new technologies. In 1985 a married New Jersey man named Bill Stern contracted with Mary Beth Whitehead to be artificially inseminated with his sperm, an arrangement that came to be known as surrogate motherhood. Bill's wife, Betsy, had multiple sclerosis, so pregnancy would have been risky for her, but this way their baby would be genetically related to one of them. Bill's contract with Whitehead called for her to give up her parental rights at a suitable time after the child's birth. Melissa Elizabeth (named Sara Elizabeth by Whitehead) was transferred to the Sterns three days after she was born, but Whitehead was already having second thoughts about the arrangement. Despondent, she threatened suicide if she wasn't allowed a visit with the baby. Concerned that she might hurt herself, the Sterns agreed. Rather than returning her to the Sterns, however, Whitehead and her husband fled to Florida where they repeatedly changed addresses to elude capture. After several months the Sterns located Whitehead and began legal proceedings to have the baby brought back to New Jersey. The ensuing custody case over "Baby M" transfixed the country. Wasn't Whitehead really the baby's mother regardless of the legal contract? Didn't she enter into the contract with the Sterns freely and fairly? The New Jersey courts did not clearly choose either of those two starkly opposed ethical positions. Instead, it decided that the child's best interests were for the Sterns to have custody, with Whitehead being granted visitation rights.

Today surrogacy contracts are still controversial, and their legal status in many states and countries is unsettled. State laws within the United States dramatically differ, as do the laws of different countries. Legalized surrogacy affords people unprecedented freedom to bring into the world healthy children who may be genetically related to their "intended parents." Mary Beth Whitehead would today be called a "traditional surrogate," as she was genetically related to the baby (as was Bill Stern). A "gestational surrogate" is not genetically related to the baby but she carries the embryo to term for the intended parents. In at least one gestational surrogacy case, where the surrogate sued for custody of the baby twins of a gay male couple, a New Jersey court in 2009 extended the *Baby M* ruling to hold the gestational surrogate to be the legal mother, despite being genetically unrelated to the children. A subsequent ruling ultimately found that custody should be awarded to the biological father. Yet considering the unsettled state of the law, as well as the evolving nature of moral views about these arrangements, this outcome was anything but predictable.

Every possible permutation of who provides what in an arrangement to bring a child into this world may now be commonly employed in surrogacy contracts. Many gay male couples provide the sperm of one partner to be used to inseminate a donor egg through IVF. Lesbian couples obtain sperm from a bank, often with substantial information about the donor's physical characteristics, or from a friend willing to be one of the biological parents with a social relationship that needs to be negotiated. Heterosexual couples where the woman faces a dangerous pregnancy often choose gestational surrogacy using both their egg and sperm.

The need for both fair and clear rules for contentious disputes over child custody is by no means unique to new reproductive technologies since divorce is estimated to mark the end of nearly half of the traditional marriages in the United States. But these new reproductive technologies inexorably multiply the number of parties who are in some position to claim child custody. In the case of gestational surrogacy, the potential claimants include two intended (contracting) parents, the egg donor, the sperm donor, and the gestational (contracting) surrogate. The ethical arguments include defending surrogacy as a consensual contract, opposing it when it unfairly exploits gestational surrogates, and opposing it unconditionally as an affront to the surrogate's dignity. Because both the unfairness and dignity arguments oppose the very use of surrogacy arrangements (conditionally versus unconditionally), neither clearly resolves what to do in the case of a custody conflict among the parties to a consummated surrogacy contract.

Both nationally and internationally, the ethical arguments for and against the practice of surrogacy show few signs of yielding a consensus about how best to resolve custody disputes. In the meantime, the use of surrogacy arrangements shows no signs of abating. Because the well-being of a child is at stake when a surrogacy contract is contested, there's every reason to place a special premium on determinate legal rules that are known to all parties before they enter into a child-creating relationship, even if those rules cannot possibly resolve the basic ethical conflicts. At stake is something far more important than a contract: the future well-being of children. (The same is true for custody disputes that occur after traditional procreation and parental divorce.) From any ethical perspective that takes seriously the basic interests of children, it's imperative to establish legal rules that protect infants from being thrown into a contentious custodial limbo. Meeting this ethical need has been a struggle within most states because citizens deeply disagree about the ethics and legality of surrogacy and other new reproductive technologies.

With the rise of gestational surrogacy arrangements that cross national borders, reconciling legal rules becomes even more challenging. Some intended parents who employ gestational surrogacy across national boundaries have found themselves in complex, drawn-out, highly publicized struggles to gain lawful recognition of their parenthood along with citizenship for the babies so conceived. When twin baby boys were born of gestational surrogacy in India in 2008, a country where surrogacy is legal and also a source of significant revenue in its "medical tourism" industry, they were stateless. The twins' intended parents, the Balazes, were citizens and residents of Germany, where surrogacy is illegal because of its potential association with eugenics. They were not recognized by their country of citizenship and residency as the legal parents of the twin boys. India had no legal obligation or intention to give citizenship to either the Balazes or their intended children. Making matters even worse, India's adoption laws blocked the Balazes from adopting the babies in India. So the two children came into the world, legally speaking, as potentially stateless orphans.

After legal appeal, an Indian High Court granted Indian citizenship to the children on humanitarian grounds, recognizing Mr. Balaz, the sperm donor and intended father, as a legal parent while recognizing the gestational surrogate as the legal mother, on grounds that she had carried the twins to term. Two years after their birth and protracted legal appeals in both India and Germany, the Balazes were allowed to adopt the twins in Germany, also on humanitarian grounds that were not intended to set a legal precedent. Without reliable legal precedents, the outcomes of reproductive contracts that cross conflicting legal boundaries remain radically uncertain.

To this day, children conceived by gestational surrogacy may be born legally stateless, parentless, or both when the intended parents reside in a country that deems surrogacy illegal and commission a gestational surrogate in another country that restricts adoption by foreign nationals. With more people making surrogacy arrangements that span national borders, just about every possible problem in determining legal parenthood has become a reality. The only constant has been the uncertainty of the outcome, which is perilous for parents and children alike. There is no sign of legal or cultural convergence across countries on how best to handle the inevitable conflicts. As legal scholar Yasmine Ergas concludes, "international commercial surrogacy appears destined to remain only loosely regulated," all but guaranteeing the "survival of conflicting legal frameworks."

EMBRYOS ON THEIR OWN

The same modern techniques that have allowed otherwise infertile couples to play the lottery have provided platforms that can help them modify it. IVF technology spread rapidly in the world of reproductive medicine. Though people like Louise Brown's parents have an enormous emotional investment in the successful production of an embryo, IVF in itself is obviously not an intimate process. For all of human history until the last fifty years, even the biological process of conception was a mystery. The very mechanism of the union of sperm and egg has only been understood since the late nineteenth century. The laboratory-located embryo is a new kind of entity in the world. The very fact that through this process the viable human embryo has a physical presence outside a uterus carries with it connotations and controversies that human beings have never faced before. That presence could be extended well beyond a few days when early-stage embryos are frozen for implantation at some later date.

A stunning example of the way biotechnology can have unanticipated consequences occurred just a few years after the birth of Louise Brown, when a California couple, Elsa and Mario Rios, died in a plane crash in Chile without having executed wills. That was in 1983. Their embryos were in Melbourne, Australia, where they had been created and preserved in 1981. Legal, ethical, and philosophical questions erupted. What to do with their two frozen embryos?

Who is responsible for them? Are they property or human beings? Is it wrong to destroy them or to use them in a medical experiment? Matters became even more unsettled when it was found that the Rios embryos were partly the product of artificial insemination. Mrs. Rios's egg was fertilized by the sperm of an anonymous donor, raising issues about the inheritance of the wealthy couple's estate. In 1987 the state government of Victoria found that the embryos did not have rights to the estate but should be thawed, and if they survived (which was deemed highly unlikely by fertility experts), they should be donated to an adoptive couple.

Another wrinkle in the social complications of IVF became visible in the case of Mary Sue and Junior Davis. Unable to conceive conventionally, seven of Mary Sue's fertilized eggs were frozen in 1988. The following year, Junior filed for divorce, but they couldn't agree about what to do with the embryos. Mary Sue wanted them initially to impregnate herself and later to donate them to another couple, but Junior preferred that they be discarded. What followed was a series of legal proceedings in which a court ruled first that the embryos were human beings whose best interest was to be brought to term, but on appeal Junior's argument that no one should be forced to become a parent prevailed. In this way uncertainties swirled around the status of the embryos. Were they persons who should be treated according to their personhood or were they property to be assigned to one party or another? Finally, in 1992 the Tennessee Supreme Court found that they were neither but had some intermediate status and that Junior Davis should not be forced to be a parent. That was the consensus legal standard until 2018, when an Arizona state law specified that frozen embryos in a custody case should go to the parent who wishes to develop them to birth, regardless of whether the other potential parent objects.

BRAVE NEW WORLDS

In an obvious sense, the new technology of reproduction doesn't "care" about whatever crisis or conflict the would-be parents are going through or where the embryo is going. Riveting legal conflicts over child custody reinforce some people's sense that these new reproductive technologies are morally dangerous. Without in any way minimizing the challenges created by new reproductive technologies, we think that it bears noting that neither does the biological reproductive process between two people "care" about the aftermath of childbirth. The norm of conceiving of and conceiving a family has long been that the biological process governs who become the parents of the child—that is, unless and until separation, divorce, or other kinds of estrangement occur, which raise familiar ethical issues unconnected to any new means of reproduction. The new reproductive technologies make us aware of some ethical questions, uncertainties, and ambiguities about parenthood and child well-being that we hadn't confronted before and that in some modalities hadn't even existed.

The birth of Louise Brown, the Rios and Davis cases, and more recently the growing popularity of IVF among gay and lesbian couples have become the backdrop for a debate that takes us beyond the goal of couples to raise a biologically related child to the question of how much control human beings should have over the likely characteristics of children. Creating embryos in laboratories not only meant that people with fertility problems or gay and lesbian couples could become parents. It also meant that those embryos could become objects of manipulation, bringing to mind images of the "fetal farm" or "Hatchery" associated with Aldous Huxley's 1932 classic and surprisingly prophetic *Brave New World*.

In Huxley's tale, the desired traits of a lower, more compliant caste could be manipulated by a vaguely described process of oxygen deprivation and alcohol exposure. Huxley knew well that ideas about improving future generations built on two thousand years of such speculation by philosophers and biologists, from Plato's ideal state in which the natural rulers try to match the best with the best, to social Darwinists who applied evolutionary theory to human society. In the twenty-first century we can hardly avoid viewing Huxley's brave new world through the lens of Nazi-style "racial improvement," and

Huxley himself portrayed his imagined world as dystopic. His novel was a satiric response to H. G. Wells and other contemporary advocates of eugenics.

Hitler's Germany decisively turned a biologically based social program advocated by progressives into a murderous ideology. But racist, nativist, and ethnocentric eugenics had plenty of precursors, including Americans who were then considered progressives. By the end of the nineteenth century, a poisonous combination of highly publicized threats to public health (symbolized in the person of Typhoid Mary, an Irish immigrant employed as a cook), and worries about the deterioration of the "American gene pool" resulted in widespread anti-immigrant sentiment that has echoes a century later. Even terrorism was in the mix after Leon Czolgosz, a Polish American "anarchist," assassinated President William McKinley in 1901. While Emma Lazarus's poem ("Give me your tired, your poor . . .") was affixed to the base of the Statue of Liberty in 1903, Congress was passing the Anarchist Exclusion Act, followed by a series of anti-immigration laws targeting southern and eastern Europeans, contributing to plummeting immigration rates in the 1930s.

Eugenics American style was by no means an entirely racist movement. Some, like activist Margaret Sanger, who founded the organization later known as Planned Parenthood, were mainly concerned about giving women control of their reproductive capacity by means of contraception in order to help them avoid poverty. Those who advocated sterilization of the "mentally defective" included among their targets many poor whites, with the tragic result that tens of thousands of Americans were sterilized. Eugenics did not need to be so ugly and hateful to be pernicious. "Better Babies" contests were originally held to call attention to infant health and mortality, but they devolved into measurements for "desirable" intellectual and physical traits that were sometimes associated with race or ethnicity.

Some of the most powerful voices were clearly racist. Among them was Madison Grant, whose highly influential tract *The Passing of the Great Race* (1916) supported the anti-immigration laws and opposed marriage between blacks and whites, all in the service of preserving the supposedly superior racial stock of northern Europe. Former Harvard biology instructor Charles Davenport, who was an advisor to the better babies movement, founded the Eugenics Records Office at Cold Spring Harbor on Long Island, New York. He argued that the social traits of various national groups could be traced to their genetic makeup, and he corresponded with proto-Nazi scientists and academic journals. Davenport's colleague at the Eugenic Records Office, Harry H. Laughlin, even received an honorary degree from the Nazified University of Heidelberg in 1936. Many pro-eugenics scientists maintained their views about social improvement through World War II. Aldous Huxley's own brother Julian, who was unlikely to be grouped with the likes of Davenport and Laughlin, advocated a "truly scientific eugenics" in his 1946 remarks as the first director general of UNESCO, the United Nations Educational, Scientific and Cultural Organization. The full picture of the mass murders and the racist ideology behind them took a while to sink in.

Aldous Huxley could not have anticipated the full-on state-sponsored racism of the Third Reich, and when he wrote his novel he didn't have access to the nature of the human genome as decoded by James Watson and Francis Crick in 1953. Geneticists immediately appreciated the implications of inserting or deleting portions of the genome, and they set about finding ways to do just that, not for eugenic purposes but to understand the basic chemistry of living things. As that goal was being approached in the early 1970s, a debate ensued between two theologians with vastly different views about the applications of the new genetics for human reproduction. That debate remains remarkably applicable today.

On one side of that debate was Joseph Fletcher, a former Episcopal priest and self-described humanist who frankly applauded the possibility that, for the first time in history, human beings could be liberated from the "reproductive roulette" that destined some for happy, healthy, successful lives and others for misery, illness, and failure. Hence the title of his 1974 book *The Ethics of Genetic*

Control, a defense of pretty much all of the measures for "improvement" that prospective parents might undertake. Fletcher's title was a direct challenge to his bête noire and the target of his arguments, the Princeton University theologian Paul Ramsey, whose 1970 book was called *Fabricated Man: The Ethics of Genetic Control*. As Ramsey surveyed the new terrain of reproductive medicine, including sperm banks and the prospects for selective breeding of human beings, he was decidedly less enthusiastic than Fletcher. Both, though, were visionaries whose debate remarkably anticipated the way two starkly opposed sides still line up today, between science enthusiasts and science skeptics. However vehement and opposed these viewpoints are, they do not precisely line up on the political left or right. Some liberals worry about the implications of already privileged people being able to gain yet more advantages for their children beyond tennis lessons and trust funds, while some conservatives identify as libertarians who decry third-party interference with parental wishes.

The role of the state is a critical background factor in historic concerns about eugenics. A key element of various pre-WWII so-called racial improvement movements was their backing by state authorities, like laws permitting involuntary sterilization. These were top-down policies to prevent certain people from reproducing while also encouraging others to do so. But even if the state's policy making was sufficient to make eugenics objectionable, was the use of state power necessary to make it so? What might be called "consumer eugenics" tests the moral significance of the state's role: What if people simply decided on their own to have, or try to have, children with or without certain qualities? Would that be morally superior and more acceptable than state-imposed conditions for having children? Consistency and coming to terms with discriminatory cultural biases set some pretty tough conditions on this view.

Science and reality add an even higher bar for eugenics, whether state or consumer based. Eugenicists' simple coupling of complex, multidimensional characteristics like intelligence to identifiable, heritable genes is nothing short of illusory. As the science journalist Carl Zimmer observes:

At the dawn of the 20th century, scientists came to limit the word *heredity* to genes. Before long, this narrow definition spread its influence far beyond genetic laboratories. It hangs like a cloud over our most personal experiences of heredity, even if we can't stop trying to smuggle the old traditions of heredity into the new language of genes. (Italics in the original.)

The qualities that a couple is likely to want their children to inherit, like intelligence, physical strength, beauty, or height are far more complex than the straightforward colored peapods of friar Gregor Mendel's genetics. They are the result of meticulous interaction among hundreds of genes and environmental triggers. So inheritance isn't about a "gene for" a certain desired quality. A little knowledge of how genetics really works can help prevent a lot of dangerous, cruel, and counterproductive politics.

Selecting embryos or even aborting fetuses based on male or female sex also doesn't sit well with many, but "family balancing" to produce a male infant when a couple already has at least one girl is seen as desirable in some cultures, especially those that value male children as more likely to provide an income for elderly parents and whose marriages don't require a dowry. Sex selection isn't a matter that falls under the heading of eugenics, but that doesn't let us off the hook of coming to terms with these and other prospective parental decisions that many people find disturbing. Some couples who both have a form of dwarfism called achondroplasia, for example, prefer to have children who can feel comfortable in their community, just as some defenders of deaf culture don't regard hearing disabilities as justifying correction by technological means.

Should certain rare choices—like short stature or deafness—be precluded against the parents' wishes because they neglect the child's best interest? The concept of child neglect may be controversial before birth, but when conception hasn't even taken place, it is still harder to apply. In any case, there are deep philosophical reasons not to tell those who are disabled what kind of children to have, as well as the fact that "disability" is a relative judgment that varies with circumstances that often are within our collective control, as when ramps and elevators are added to buildings and antidiscrimination policies are implemented. Modern societies have come to appreciate a responsibility to provide reasonable opportunities for everyone to participate in the life of the commons.

CONSUMER EUGENICS?

With authoritarian eugenics largely in the rearview mirror by the end of the twentieth century, a small consumer eugenics industry began to fascinate the public far beyond its scale. A sperm donor industry offered semen from well-educated young men whose square-jawed images spoke volumes about a desirable type. Couples advertised for egg donors with certain characteristics, especially tall, Ivy League–educated women. Ethnic preferences also abound: opportunity prevails in ads for Jewish and Korean ova, for example. LGBTQ (lesbian, gay, bisexual, transgender, queer/questioning) couples are increasingly interested in assisted reproduction that enables them to have a genetically related child, by selecting either a man for their sperm donor or a woman for their egg donation. These couples also may make donor decisions based on certain desired characteristics.

It's commonplace now for singles of marital disposition to post online their detailed preferences for dates who they hope to become their mates. It's no great leap to understanding infertile couples' seeking their desired genetic traits in offspring. Whatever misgivings we have about specific traits actively sought in spouses or children, these need to be squared with our attitude toward age-old practices of selective mating by choice for the purposes of procreation. Online and social media advertising combined with new procreative technologies have added considerably more precision and publicity to these choices. DNA profiles can easily be posted on dating sites, allowing prospective mates to assess genetic potential in ways that feel more science based than judgments based on physical appearance.

The prospective end of what Joseph Fletcher called genetic roulette has led some to worry about its implications for that most familiar expectation of parenthood: we will love and cherish the results of the roll of the genetic dice regardless of what comes up. What if the product isn't what was ordered? Few human characteristics are genetically simple enough to be controlled by a single gene. The vast majority of traits, especially those involving intellect and personality, are the result of a delicate interplay of genes and environment that may be so complex as to resist ever being managed and certainly will not be in the foreseeable future. Considering the virtual impossibility of "designer babies," we need to take seriously the potential psychological damage to children who fail to make some expected grade. The number of unloved, neglected, or abused children is already far too great. There's not enough experience with these practices to know whether their record would be worse than for children born from traditional reproduction. Parental expectations from the "natural lottery" may also be unrealistic.

The most accurate "warning" label that can be placed for the foreseeable future on all human reproduction: most of the outcome of your actions will be subject to a reproductive lottery. This is true for both the traditional and the technologically sophisticated means of conceiving a child. And it's consistent with the choices future parents make that have some effect in influencing a small proportion of the results of their reproduction.

THE NEW NATURAL LAW

Reproductive lotteries are not in any mathematical sense close to purely random. Typically overlooked in debates over "designer babies" is the fact that the traditional mating patterns resulting in traditional reproduction have not been remotely random. Even before the invention of precisely targeted online apps with their detailed online questionnaires for finding prospective spouses, couples very selectively met and mated. Whether it was arranged marriages that used tight familial social networks or modern marriages premised on romantic attraction, most prospective spouses have long sought their mates, whether consciously or not, among those with similar social backgrounds. What's different is that mates traditionally exercised no control over the results of their subsequent reproduction. That is the so-called genetic lottery. But there is no evidence that the children conceived through the new reproductive technologies are less loved than those conceived in the traditional way. Considering that the children brought into the world through new reproductive technologies are at least as badly wanted as any others, we suspect that most of these children will continue to be fortunate indeed.

We still would do well to consider unanticipated social ramifications to these new ways of making babies. We begin by observing that no a priori reason exists to assume from the untraditional or unnatural nature of new procreative technologies that they are unethical. Or that the children born of these technologies are loved less deeply or cared for any less well than others. Nonetheless, ever since the advent of IVF, and indeed since the appearance of the birth control pill, the social implications of separating sex and reproduction from monogamous relationships between men and women have been cause for serious concerns. The bioethicist Leon Kass has mourned the extinction of traditional courtship and family relations in the developed world, a major social change he sees made more likely (or at the very least reinforced) by modern reproductive technologies. On this view the nuclear family founded on romantic love and marriage is a precious and fragile institution. Kass is also among those social conservatives, including legal theorist Robert George, whose views extend what's called the "natural law" tradition, one that dates back to Aristotle.

The modernized New Natural Law holds that the most fundamental moral values, including those related to love, sex, and reproduction, take precedence over human-made law. These fundamental values require reference both to the relevant human emotional capacities and physical organs that were naturally created and to the ethical precepts that are knowable through the exercise of our reason. The New Natural Law claims that "spouses unite bodily only by coitus [sexual intercourse], which is ordered toward the good of bringing new human life into the world." Marriage that is "sealed or consummated: in coitus, which is organic bodily union," also is said to uniquely capture the true (human to human) love:

> Marriage is ordered to family life because the act by which spouses make love also makes new life, one and the same act both seals a marriage and brings forth children. That is why marriage alone is the loving union of mind and body fulfilled by the procreation—and rearing—of whole new human beings.

In this view, over time any disruption of that traditional "natural" system undermines the precious social arrangements that go with it, including the traditional family composed of a man, a woman, and their children. In his trenchant critique of this position, political theorist Stephen Macedo pinpoints its crux: "no coitus, no marriage."

The New Natural Law draws inferences from the structure and function of human genitalia that defy both logic and ethics. It degrades respectable differences in sexual orientations and preferences among human beings, rendering it unnatural and therefore (in a leap of logic) unethical for LGBTQ individuals to have sexual relationships, let alone to use reproductive arrangements such as surrogacy to become loving parents. Natural law analysis also once justified laws against interracial marriage on the grounds that such marriages were unnatural. Moreover, from antiquity to our own time, people have turned out to be much more adaptable and variable in finding and making meaning in their lives than these renderings of natural law suggest. Over the millennia, many families have flourished that have not been formed in accordance with the natural law stereotype. Cousin marriage remains common in many traditional cultures. New reproductive technologies have offered LGBTQ parents a newfound freedom to conceive and raise children whom they will love and care for. Consistent with that freedom, new kinds of families consisting of loving same-sex parents are more common—and more public—than ever.

REMEMBER THE FUTURE

The particular individuals who will or will not be conceived as a result of reproductive decisions are of course absent from that decision making, and not just because they don't yet exist. It's also because we cannot possibly know who they will be until they are conceived, and countless contingencies change the specific self who comes into existence when we procreate. This means that our sense of responsibility for future people and generations transcends the notion of obligations to specific future individuals. When we collectively care about the well-being of future people and generations, without knowing their particular identities, we share an ethical sensibility that is well adapted to the human reproductive lottery on a macro scale. In a sense, this is a "cosmic" sensibility. Future children, people, and generations, whoever they turn out to be, are the objects of our responsibility for the future. For a meaningful start, we may want to try to ensure that their opportunities to live a healthy life are at least as good as our own.

An ethics of responsibility means that to care about future people and generations, we don't need to be obligated to identifiable future people. Every decent society acts on some such assumption of responsibility for the well-being of future generations. We can think of our ethical responsibility as directed toward making the future a healthy one for whoever happens to be born. Our ethical acts directed toward the future are analogous in this way to how we approach the reproductive lottery of life. We cannot possibly predetermine the identities of those who will be the future beneficiaries of even our most deliberate, carefully planned actions. Yet we should do our part to ensure that whoever they turn out to be, their opportunities in life turn out to be at least as good as ours.

No society rejects the idea of responsibility for the well-being of future generations, partly because no clear line can be drawn between one generation and another. Most people care about ensuring a decent life for their progeny. Even though this sense of caring is familial, because of the nature of the reproductive lottery, it's not an obligation toward particular individuals since it's directed toward generations that have yet to be conceived. We can defend it as a sense of responsibility toward future generations and also as our obligation to many actual others, present and past, who by their own good deeds have contributed to our well-being. This future-oriented way of recognizing our debt to others who came before us often goes by the maxim "pay it forward."

Many significant social enterprises are consistent with this profound sense of moral responsibility to provide benefits to future persons even though we can't know who the particular individuals will turn out to be. Some agricultural systems are designed to produce benefits over many decades and even hundreds of years to future generations. Some great construction projects require decades to complete. Many cathedrals require generation upon generation of consuming commitment for their realization. Barcelona's Segrada Família church is an awe-inspiring extreme, construction having begun in 1882 and not expected to be completed until 2026, the centenary of the death of its chief architect, Antoni Gaudí. These projects pay homage to the idea that despite the fact that none of us can know who in particular will inhabit the future, we may want to do our part for the benefit of future people and generations, whoever they might be.

DISEASE PREVENTION

Is it possible to be more specific about our responsibility to future persons and generations than these general observations suggest? We can begin by specifying some minimum conditions that are largely uncontroversial and protect newborns against the most serious, life-threatening liabilities that would otherwise result from a reproductive lottery. For example, newborns should be screened for serious disease. The screening process has to involve very low if any risk, it can disclose certain conditions generally regarded as posing serious risks, and interventions need to be available that can eliminate or greatly reduce the harmful effects of the disease. Current policies largely follow those guidelines. All U.S. states routinely screen every newborn according to those criteria. Although policies vary from state to state, most screen for a few dozen conditions that include phenylketonuria, cystic fibrosis, sickle cell disease, hearing loss, and congenital heart disease. Only a few drops of blood are required.

Routine newborn screening doesn't meet any definition of eugenics because the goal is to identify treatable disorders, not to eliminate alternative forms of a gene. Though some parents with hearing loss might complain that screening for hereditary deafness is a form of discrimination, hardly anyone objects to being prepared to create the best possible circumstances for their child to thrive. Therefore, even though governments are involved, state systems to provide newborn screening fall within the ambit of obligations to future persons without being considered eugenic.

Setting aside prenatal testing for medical reasons, what we have called consumer eugenics carries echoes of systematic selection for certain traits, and it risks the moral taint of historical experience. But even if many couples decide to try to aggressively shape their child's genetic future in detail—an enterprise that is sure to disappoint them given the realities of the way genes interact and are shaped by their environment—human beings don't reproduce prodigiously enough to make for widespread genetic changes in the species for centuries to come. The same is not true for rapidly propagating species like insects. A few mosquito reproductive cycles can cause genes to be passed on to millions of individual mosquitoes, so ideas like causing sterility to prevent a population from spreading diseases like malaria are provocative but carry uncertain risks for the ecosystem. As we learn more about the basic science of living things, we learn more about the limitations of old ideas about perfect babies. At the same time, new genetic technologies present far more targeted and efficient ways to modify the molecules that manage heredity than ever before.

Preventing disease in future children does not count, even remotely, as a pernicious form of eugenics, but changing genes in human embryos, especially if they can be inherited, is part of the array of disease-preventing reproductive technologies made possible by IVF now on the horizon. The implications of these technologies do call for serious bioethical consideration. A prime example is the combination of benefits and tradition-bending medical technology that has provoked an intense international bioethics debate about mitochondrial replacement therapy (MRT), which can prevent babies from being born with a group of serious diseases. In a female embryo, once that inheritance is prevented, it permanently changes some of the genes of all female descendants. It also involves three biological parents. The combination of technological change of a line of descent and the idea of a "three-parent embryo" has been enough to cause many to wonder if the likely benefits are on balance worthwhile.

The medical problem lies in the mitochondria, a small energy-producing cellular organ that in human beings contains thirty-seven genes, in addition to the roughly twenty thousand genes in the cell's nucleus. Sometimes these genes mutate and are associated with a wide range of neurological and other disorders. Treatments are limited, but the very precise tools of reproductive technology make it possible for at-risk embryos to be "engineered" so that they will not be affected. In principle the idea is remarkably simple. When a prospective mother might transmit a mitochondrial disorder to a future child, the nucleus of her egg cell is removed in the IVF clinic and placed in a donor egg with healthy mitochondria that has had its nucleus removed. The resulting egg cell is then fertilized with sperm. The resulting embryo is not at risk of mitochondrial disease and can be brought to term as usual in the mother's uterus. Technically the embryo has three parents: the woman whose nuclear DNA was transferred to the donor egg, the egg donor (though that amounts to a tiny percentage of the baby's genes), and the man who contributed his sperm. Only two of the "technical" parents intend to become the legally recognized, loving, and caregiving parents.

In 2016 committees in both the United States and the United Kingdom gave cautious green lights for mitochondrial replacement therapy, though the U.S. group limited MRT for the time being to male embryos because they will not pass mitochondria on to future children. As confidence and public comfort with the procedure grows, that stricture may well be dropped. For all the heightened concerns about "designer babies" raised by the new reproductive technologies, MRT also drives home an important and enduring lesson: when it comes to the characteristics and character of children, we are increasingly able to anticipate preventing some inheritable diseases but we are nowhere near being able to predict let alone willing and able to control the myriad genetic and environmental results of human reproductive lotteries.

MRT reengineers human embryos to minimize the chances of a child being born with a set of deadly diseases. If many women who would otherwise be at high risk of bearing children with mitochondrial diseases end up using what's found to be safe MRT procedures, these children's parents will be engaging in what is essentially still a reproductive lottery. It is a purposively reengineered lottery, to be sure. But as certainly, these reengineered human reproductive lotteries overwhelmingly defy any predetermined plan of who our children will be. While new reproductive technologies are significantly altering specific components of the lottery of human birth, they do not, and we think they should not, alter this most basic recipe for responsible parenthood and sane parenting: to relish the unpredictable characteristics and character of our children, and to love them for their perfect imperfection.

Nine

OPENING CELL DOORS

Nothing is more obvious about our bodies than that they are so variegated—not one undifferentiated whole but divided into diverse parts. Human beings have taken millennia to figure out the functions of these parts, and we are still very far from a complete account of the way our bodies work. There have been lots of eddies and blind alleys along the way. Though the roles of large solid organs like the liver, kidney, and pancreas are now fairly well understood, the truth is that we are still unsure about the functions of many of our smaller pieces, and even less sure about how they work together. And in some cases, like the gut flora that make up what's called our microbiome, we've only recently realized how clueless we are about all the ways our parts interact. Technology has played an absolutely essential role in getting us as far as we have come, as when philosopher-scientist Robert Hooke looked through his microscope in the seventeenth century and saw tiny structures in cork. He called them cells because they reminded him of a monk's Spartan living quarters.

IMMORTAL LINES

It turned out that Hooke's so-called cells were a reasonable place for modern biology to start. More than two hundred different kinds of cells make up the adult human body. As objects of investigation, cells satisfy the Goldilocks' maxim: they are neither too big nor too little, but just right. They are, for one thing, constituents of every organ.

It stands to reason that if we could understand how they work both separately and together, and if we could prevent them from going wrong, we could avoid or correct the conditions of our larger systems that we call "disease." When we are diseased, our options have traditionally been limited to watchful waiting, symptom management, relatively low-tech interventions like physical therapy or talk therapy, and drugs, radiation, or surgery. All of these options are limited in their direct effectiveness, time efficiency, avoidance of serious side effects, or all three. They may also be quite expensive and require more treatment later.

Treating our cells directly would not only give us another option but perhaps also one that restores us without the need for long-term follow-up. If we could go beyond keeping those cells functioning well by even improving some of them, we might be able to push out the boundaries of what is possible for creatures like ourselves. With the ability to manipulate cells and their parts comes a challenging question: Under what conditions is it ethical to do so?

At a basic level, the crucial role of cells in the life sciences was vividly documented in the story of Henrietta Lacks, an African American woman who worked as a tobacco farmer, raised five children, and died at age thirty-one of cervical cancer in 1951 in the "colored" ward of the only major Baltimore hospital (at Johns Hopkins University) that would admit blacks. The cells from her cervical cancer tumor were proven to be so resilient that they were made into an "immortal" cell line that was used in historically important, life-saving experiments, including those that led to the first polio vaccine. Historian Rebecca Skloot's riveting history of Lacks's "immortal life" raises troubling questions about the role of racism and disrespect for individuals, their families, and their communities, as well as what equitable treatment requires in the practice of medicine and life sciences research.

Twenty-five years after Henrietta Lacks's death, John Moore's cancerous spleen was removed at UCLA Medical Center. The protein in Moore's blood cells turned out to be useful for products that could stimulate white blood cell growth and improve resistance to infections. The cells from Moore's spleen would have been discarded as medical waste, as stipulated in the consent form he signed. For years Moore agreed to additional samples being taken from other parts of his body, until a new consent form mentioned potential products that could be developed from his blood or bone marrow. When Moore sued on the grounds that he should share in any potential profits, the courts ultimately found that he had no property rights but that Moore's doctor should have disclosed his financial interest.

Much knowledge has been gained and much suffering has been prevented through the use of the derivatives of cells from the bodies of Lacks, Moore, and many other patients, and substantial portions and profits of the pharmaceutical industry have been based on them. Yet the original "HeLa" cells were obtained in 1951 without Lacks's or her family's knowledge. Repeatedly since that time and as recently as 2013, the privacy of Lacks and her family was violated by researchers and journalists who made her medical records and her family's genetic history public. The stories of Henrietta Lacks and John Moore both emphasize what people in their position actually expect and what they surely should be entitled to: transparency and privacy. Every major advance in the life sciences demands that we improve our individual and collective understandings well beyond the more abstract matters of science and ethics.

DISCOVERING STEM CELLS

For decades peculiar tumors called teratomas had occasionally been found in ovaries and testicles. The presence of hair and bone in those places was curious if not downright shocking, but it gave rise to a hunch that has more than borne out: those out-of-place tissues must be the erroneous products of the potent cells that later produce all of the various specialized cells in the body. Somehow their genetic instructions went wrong while the reproductive organs were being formed. That error suggested that it might be possible to obtain the precursor or "stem" cells from early embryos that gave rise to all the later kinds of body cells, as well as the sperm and egg cells.

Obtaining those embryonic stem cells and studying them in the laboratory wouldn't only be a matter of scientific curiosity. The information about how they differentiate could also help us understand how and why some fetuses don't survive or why others survive with serious anomalies. Another promising idea was that those stem cells could be modified so that for people with heart disease, for example, their own healthy heart muscle stem cells could be implanted to treat the illness. Using a person's own cells would also avoid the problem of immune rejection. That would be personalized, stem cell-based medicine.

The path to following up on those ambitious ideas required that first step: isolating human embryonic stem cells in a laboratory. That feat was accomplished by two labs in 1998, one led by James Thomson at the University of Wisconsin and another by John Gearhart, then at Johns Hopkins University. The path to learning what those cells can teach us was indeed entrancing, but matters weren't so simple. In order to obtain those embryonic stem cells, they had to be removed from a donated human embryo that was about six days old, which in turn meant its destruction. Or stem cells could be derived from tissues of aborted five- to nine-week-old fetuses. The ensuing controversy led to a decade-long debate in bioethics and an unprecedented public feud among bioethicists who had conflicting views about the beginning of life. Their conflicts bore a family resemblance to the even more divisive ones between pro-life and pro-choice advocates over abortion that for decades and to this very day embroil American politics. When grouped together (often loosely but fervently) by critics with deeply divided opinions over the nature of family, the role of women, and the significance of racial and ethnic identities in public life, these controversies came to be called the "culture wars."

Even before the controversy over using embryonic stem cells broke out in 1998, the ground for a major public bioethics debate was stoked by another milestone. In 1996 a group of Scottish veterinarians cloned a nonhuman mammal, a sheep they called Dolly (briefly mentioned in chapter 2). Dolly had been produced by taking an unfertilized egg cell from one kind of sheep with a white face, removing the nucleus with most of the DNA, replacing it with the nucleus of a mammary cell from a sheep with a black face, then putting the new "embryo" into a sheep uterus to give birth. The result, Dolly, had a white face that proved it was the genetic product of the nucleus from the second sheep and not that of the sheep egg cell.

The scientists' goal was to prove a principle about improving breeding stock, but they also created a firestorm well beyond their limited purpose: If one kind of mammal can be cloned, then why not human beings? And what exactly would that mean? Reproductive human cloning stimulated fears about creepy scenarios that would further upset traditional family relationships, like a grieving husband who might want to use his late wife's DNA to produce a female child with an egg donor so that the baby would be a "copy" of his wife, then adopt the baby and raise her as his daughter. While many worried about how reproductive cloning would further undermine traditional values, others celebrated the idea that human clones could herald a new dawn of superhumans. One group announced, without evidence, that they had cloned a person in order to establish a path to human immortality. So far the promised clones have not appeared.

The very notion of a clone as a copy of the original is misleading. With the exception of only a few traits, what we become is determined by the interaction of genes with the environment. That gene-environment interaction begins with the womb itself. There were reassurances that cloned humans would be distinct individuals, that they would not necessarily resemble the "original," and that a clone would be less similar to the person whose nuclear DNA was obtained than an identical twin would be to the twin (because not all DNA is in the nucleus). And from a practical ethical standpoint, even to attempt to clone a human being would be very dangerous for the mother and the fetus because it took hundreds of attempts to achieve Dolly's birth. (The first successful cloning of primates, in 2018, those being macaque monkeys, also involved a high failure rate as reported by the team in China.) All these facts were less than central to the remarkable amount of public comment and fascination that Dolly stimulated. In 1997, with the chair of his bioethics commission, Harold Shapiro, at his side, President Clinton announced a ban on the use of federal funds for research on human cloning.

Two years after Dolly's birth, when the isolation of human embryonic stem cells was announced, the excitement and confusion about the meaning of cloning was still simmering. It didn't take long for the stem cell research issue to meld with the cloning controversy, raising larger questions about how far reproductive biology and bioengineering could go and should be allowed to go. These were not new questions—they have loomed large in Western culture at least since Mary Shelley's *Frankenstein* was published in 1818—but by the time those embryonic stem cells were isolated in the University of Wisconsin and the Johns Hopkins University labs, the conversation explicitly entered politics. Major party presidential candidates felt great pressure to weigh in on the issue. After the smoke cleared in the legally contested 2000 election, President George W. Bush held a series of earnest Oval Office conversations with philosophers and theologians during the summer of 2001. Following those reflections, the first of their kind in any presidency, Bush declared that he would permit no more federal funding for research on the cells of human embryos destroyed after that date, but that research involving cells from previously destroyed embryos could continue. The president also announced that he would form a bioethics council to advise him on issues in biomedical science and technology.

Initial reaction to the president's stem cell funding policy was mixed. At first, many scientists welcomed the opportunity to continue to work with at least some of the cells, and many conservatives and some liberals appreciated that the president was drawing an ethical line of sorts. Gradually, though, many in the scientific community worried about the symbolism of any constraints on funding research that involved embryos that were created by IVF in a laboratory, that were donated with full consent, and that would never have been used to create a pregnancy. For them, the issue was bigger than stem cell science itself; it extended to suspicion about the Bush administration's attitude toward science in general. These concerns were reinforced by the dominant philosophical orientation of the members of the president's bioethics council. The chair, Leon Kass, was a trenchant critic of what he regarded as a tendency for both innovative biology and its progressive supporters to undermine moral traditions. Under his leadership, the bioethics council advocated and sought to model what he called a "richer bioethics," which meant, among other things, one not so favorably disposed to new technological possibilities and the changing nature of the family.

POTENT POLITICS

Though bioethicists had found themselves swept up in political debates about issues like abortion and euthanasia before, the stem cell controversy took matters to a new level. In earlier decades, doubts were raised about doctors' willingness to engage in practices that aimed to end a pregnancy or cut short a human life. This time the moral integrity of scientists themselves was in question and their willingness to use or endorse the use of products of a laboratory technique—deriving cells from embryos—that involved the destruction of a handful of human embryos that would never otherwise have been brought to term. Biologists protested that their goal was to understand basic science and ultimately to produce new medical treatments. States like California and New York responded by committing public funds to stem cell biology, while some other states put up roadblocks to the field. Scientists who had not previously been involved in political issues found themselves signing petitions, writing editorials, meeting with state officials, and making career decisions based on states that seemed more science-friendly than others.

At about the same time, some climate scientists were also drawn into political arguments when they were accused of misrepresenting the threat of climate change. This was more than a coincidence. Surveys show that since the late 1970s, self-identified conservatives have lost confidence in some fields of science. Those results are consistent with many studies indicating a general diminishing confidence in established institutions. This is a change from the pre–Vietnam War and Watergate days, when the dominant science story was the space program, capped by the moon landing in 1969. Events like the Karen Ann Quinlan case, the advent of recombinant DNA (rDNA), and the birth of "test-tube baby" Louise Brown shifted Americans' attention from physics and engineering to the promise and perils of the life sciences. Developments in experimental biology have often been drawn into the heated environment of debates about abortion and contraception. All touch on the fraught question of the moral status of a human embryo. As Kass observed, surrounded by issues like cloning and stem cells, we are all living in embryoville.

Despite President Bush's limitations on research funding, research involving human embryonic stem cells continued. Yet there were still few rules about what studies could be done ethically, assuming that not all research with the embryonic cell lines was necessarily unethical, and how it could be done. Reminded of the way that the scientific community took control of public worries and political reactions to early DNA engineering in the 1970s, some science leaders thought it important for scientists to develop standards for lab work with the cells. An obvious venue was the National Academy of Sciences, which was chartered in 1863 by the Lincoln administration to provide advice on science. In 2005 an academy committee made a series of recommendations concerning research on embryos donated by a couple with their informed consent and without payment for the embryos. No embryos would be created only for science. The guidelines also set strict rules about putting human stem cells into nonhuman animals, which directly addressed concerns about "humanized" animals.* For the opponents of the research, any science that treated

---

* Jonathan was co-chair of this committee.

human embryos as products disposable for research, however important, was unacceptable. President Bush aligned himself with an effort to urge couples planning on pregnancy via IVF to adopt embryos left over in fertility clinics, dubbed "snowflake babies."

BETWEEN THE LINES

Despite its political resonance and association with the culture wars, the controversy about human embryonic stem cells didn't line up as a simple split between liberals and conservatives or pro-choice versus pro-life. Liberals who were generally pro-science nonetheless worried that new treatments from stem cell biology would be available only to the wealthy. Some conservatives and some libertarians decried any actions by government that created obstacles to freedom of thought and scientific inquiry. Underlying these cross-currents were fundamental questions about the power of science in the modern world in relation to the human self, which have only grown more complicated over time and are by no means limited to the stem cell issue alone. Important medical research often involves putting some human cells into animals to test the cells under various conditions. These lab models, usually rodents, are called "chimera," after a creature in Greek mythology made up of recognizable body parts of several different animals—often a lion, a goat, and a snake.

Ethics in the care of patients, experimental subjects, and animals had long been on the public mind when President George W. Bush marked yet another bioethics milestone in his 2006 State of the Union Address. The president urged Congress "to pass legislation to prohibit the most egregious abuses of medical research." This time, rather than concerns about widespread vaccination studies or drug trials in dying patients or the abuse of animals, the issue was the blurring of lines between species. President Bush opposed "human-animal hybrids" in which the genes of two different species are fused. Then-Senator Sam Brownback introduced the Human-Animal Hybrid Prohibition Act of 2009. If passed, the bill would have prohibited the creation of a whole range of human-nonhuman organisms as "grossly unethical" because they "blur the line between human and animal, male and female, parent and child, and one individual and another individual." Congress never passed the bill, but two state legislatures, Arizona and Louisiana, did create laws with language similar to Brownback's bill.

Why did these esoteric lab experiments rise to the level of presidential concern, and what is the point of such studies? The underlying worry was that creating lab animals with a mixture of human and nonhuman parts undermines human dignity, regardless of the important scientific purpose of the research. (There are also some deep philosophical questions here, such as whether species per se have a moral status or are first and foremost convenient classifications.) Biologists sometimes talk about "humanizing" some feature of an animal, but that's typically shorthand for a modification, often genetic, that enables isolating and studying one particular function that cannot ethically or practically be studied in humans. How, for example, to regrow ears for children who have lost theirs in accidents or because of disease? Pictures of a human ear grown on the back of a rodent have been on internet sites as examples of creepy science, but the children who would ultimately receive such grafts and their parents would surely be grateful for them. Animal models like the ones those bills sought to ban are also basic tools for studying cell biology so that cells might someday replace damaged tissue, like brain cells for addressing Parkinson's disease and stroke. For decades, research on diseases like AIDS and leukemia included human-mouse bone marrow transplants. Our experience, backed up by survey evidence, has been that when people understand the purpose of conducting research with human-animal hybrids, they overwhelmingly agree that it should continue.

A SCIENTIFIC SOLUTION?

Just as soon as embryonic stem cells were isolated from early embryos and aborted fetuses in the laboratory in 1998, close observers of the ensuing controversy about their use in research knew that alternatives to embryonic stem cells were technically feasible. It took less than ten years for that alternative to be developed—a fairly rapid clip in the world of biology. The general idea was to expose an adult's cells to certain genes that would signal the DNA in the cells to turn back into their potent original state, before they became specialized as certain kinds of body cells. It was a matter of exposing the adult cells to various combinations of genes until the right signals were identified. In 2007 a Japanese lab reported that a combination of only four genes had that effect in human cells. They were called induced pluripotent stem cells: "induced" because they were the result of modifying adult cells, and "pluripotent" because of their potential to become the many varied body cells. With this new tool, asking questions about what could be done with very potent cells might not require the use of embryonic cells, thereby avoiding all the controversy they entailed.

Many labs immediately turned away from embryonic to induced pluripotent cells, which are easier to manage and to grow, though they might be less useful for some research purposes. Embryonic stem cells remain the "gold standard" of potency that pluripotent cells are measured against, and they remain in use for some experiments. Perhaps the most immediate benefits of pluripotent stem cells were for public officials who found themselves eager to support science but who also wanted to respect the special moral status that embryos are widely granted. The results of the Japanese work gave Senator John McCain some room to bring apparently clashing values closer together at a crucial moment when he was running for president against then-Senator Barack Obama in 2008. Asked in one of the Republican primary debates about banning the use of human embryonic stem cells, a position staunchly held by many conservatives, McCain—a strong opponent of abortion rights—did not advocate an outright ban. Nancy Reagan was especially concerned about the usefulness of embryonic stem cells in researching Alzheimer's disease, which had afflicted her beloved husband, President Ronald Reagan, for over a decade before his death. McCain had also pointed out in a Republican primary debate that "these stem cells are either going to be discarded or perpetually frozen." But he added that he hoped for the usefulness instead of pluripotent stem cells derived from adult cells.

When Barack Obama took office, the relative advantages of embryonic or pluripotent stem cells remained unsettled. He allowed federal funding for research on many more lines of stem cells derived from human embryos. But at the same time, he deferred to Congress about precluding the use of federal money for the process that led to the destruction of the embryos to obtain the cells. Both McCain and Obama—one from a more conservative and the other from a more liberal starting point—found ways of lessening the clash between the pursuit of potentially lifesaving science and the protection of human embryos that no public official could eliminate.

Despite continuing arguments among scientists about the limits of pluripotent stem cells, ongoing research has demonstrated that they can be quite useful. One example is an understanding of the mechanism of the Zika virus, which could open a pathway to preventing the condition in infants. In another example, induced pluripotent stem cells are being developed to replace the brain cells that fail to produce a chemical called dopamine, the underlying cause of Parkinson's disease. Researchers hope to be able to use the patient's own cells for this transformation and that the body's immune system won't reject them as foreign tissue.

With some distance from the embryonic stem cell controversy, the evidence is now overwhelming both that induced pluripotent stem cells are useful in many experiments and that cells from embryos made it possible to get there. History teaches us that, for all its accompanying uncertainty and controversy, such basic research has no close substitute to advance the prospects for better treatment, prevention, and cure for the countless millions of individuals and families worldwide who will be afflicted by Alzheimer's, Parkinson's, and other neurodegenerative diseases.

DEAD CELLS REBORN

By the early 2000s the field of bioethics, though still engaged in patient care problems, had completed a turn toward ethical issues in the basic laboratory sciences. This trend was greatly influenced by the scale and implications of the human genome project and the public interest that it generated. No sooner had some resolution come to the stem cell debate than new experimental results opened up another debate about engineering cells.

In 2010 the J. Craig Venter Institute in Maryland announced that his group had reengineered a cell using a synthetic genome. Taking a made-from-scratch length of DNA, humanly engineered from its chemical parts, the Venter group had transplanted it into a bacterium, *Mycoplasma capricolum*. Within a few dozen cell divisions, the synthetic DNA had taken over the cell's functions, all traces of its original genome had disappeared, and the cell was self-replicating. This remarkable accomplishment in a field that has come to be known as synthetic biology, or "synbio" for short, immediately excited pronouncements about its scientific and ethical significance. There was no doubt that a cellular engineering milestone had been reached. Some went so far as to declare that Venter is the first scientist to truly play God, an ambiguous assertion (taken at its best) that wasn't vigorously disputed by Venter. That sensationalist description was accompanied, predictably, by demands that synthetic genomics research cease and desist and that, if necessary, there should be a government ban on it.

On the same day that Venter announced this breakthrough, with worldwide media coverage, President Obama asked his Presidential Commission for the Study of Bioethical Issues, as its first order of business, to review the benefits, risks, and "appropriate ethical boundaries" of this new field, and to present him with its findings before year's end. Those public deliberations gave voice to the widest range of viewpoints, from "let this science rip" without regulation to "ban this risky research" until its risks are clearly identified and mitigated. With an overarching aim of *earning* public trust in the integrity of both the scientific and engineering communities and the applicable regulatory systems"—and the shared conviction that what's at stake was everybody's business—the commission held open deliberations that gave voice to the critiques as well as aspirations of this new biotechnology.

The deliberations began by considering synthetic biology's potential benefits because without any credible promise of benefits, no risks would be worth taking. These include drug and vaccine development that is quicker, less costly, and less dependent on scarce natural products. The plant extract that's the basis for treating malaria, for example, can be semisynthesized, potentially providing reliable, affordable, first-line treatment for a disease that's estimated to kill nearly half a million people, mostly young children, each year. Algae and other microbes may be synthetically engineered to create more efficient and cleaner-burning fuels. The air we breathe and water we drink can be made cleaner and safer if synthetic biology realizes its potential. So there's a lot at stake on the upside, however uncertain this potential may be.

The major objections to synthetic biology turned out to be of two kinds. The first is that the application of this technique significantly aggravates threats of both *bio-error*, enabling some unintended environmental threat, and *bioterror*, the hostile use of bioengineering. The second objection is that, in creating or even attempting to create some altered form of life partly from nonlife (in this case, a string of chemicals arranged as base pairs), a fundamental line has been breached, that "God-playing" in the laboratory has finally and truly arrived. As two medical ethicists put their critique, "seen from the perspective of synthetic biology, nature is a blank space to be filled with whatever we wish." Is this then the ultimate human hubris, humankind recklessly lording it over nature?

The first aggravated threat objection has some significant merit, the commission found, though not as much as is often claimed, at least not in the short- or midterm, and the threat is not unique to synthetic biology. The possibility of human error will need to be addressed, as always, through education, and also through cultural change among scientists, in addition to well-established systems of accountability and record keeping that expand to include synthetic biologists. While there's scant evidence to claim that Venter's experiment is "the quintessential Pandora's box moment," as it was called by one critic of biotechnology, developing the technology presents some serious risks. A synthetic organism might inadvertently be released from a lab, for example, and multiply in environmentally destructive ways. This example is especially instructive because synthetic biology also has great positive potential for engineering microbes that could advance clean-burning fuels and bioremediation as well as help to contain climate change.

The second objection to the cell reboot was that Venter and his colleagues had played God by creating synthetic life, thereby crossing a moral line. This critique of new science and technology has been heard many times before. In the case of the Venter group's work, however, no less a theological authority than the Vatican pronounced synthetic biology acceptable if used to treat disease and clean up the environment. One official of the Italian bishops' conference still took the opportunity to issue a reminder that scientists "should never forget there is only one creator: God."

A general unease remains that synthetic biologists will be reckless or even intentional and nonbenevolent in imposing their untrammeled will over nature. So let's be clear: for synthetic biology, or any science or biotechnology, to be an ethical enterprise, its practitioners must not treat our natural world as "a blank space to be filled with whatever we [or they] wish." Eminent biologists, like Bonnie Bassler, who testified before the commission, are among the most passionate and clearheaded in arguing that—precisely because we understand such a small fraction of the biological world and the evolution of organisms has been long in the making—the notion of imposing our "wishes" upon a "blank space" is the ultimate hubris. It's as foolish as it would be unethical.

Such hubris should not be confused with a very different idea that comes with the territory of our being *Homo sapiens* and that drives not only the life sciences and engineering but also the social sciences and humanities at their best: we try to understand and help improve the world, which importantly includes nature. The commission's report therefore called attention to the fact that:

> Biological systems have developed over billions of years, and their interactions with the environment are astoundingly complex. We are far from being proficient speakers of the language of life, and our capacity to control synthetic organisms that we design and release into the world is promising but unproven.

The commission concluded its public deliberations with a call for "prudent vigilance" to secure three social values: the *intellectual freedom* of synthetic biologists as they seek to realize the potential *public benefits* of revolutionary technologies, but with established oversight mechanisms that monitor and mitigate risks over time to ensure *responsible stewardship of our planet*.

BIG DATA

Infusing a person with synthetic molecules—unnatural molecules that have been humanly engineered with a disarmed virus—once may have sounded like the stuff of science fiction, and to many people it still may sound that way. It's quite the opposite of treating nature as an empty slate, however, since it starts with a cancer patient's own cells. And, as far as we can fathom, it's no more "playing God" than any humanly manufactured medicine, but this medicine happens to be a living drug. It's the revolutionary approach of adoptive cell transfer (ACT), which collects and then reengineers a patient's own immune cells to treat some of the deadliest cancers (a treatment that is generally called immunotherapy).

CAR-T therapy is one type of ACT. The CAR-T cells essential to this immunotherapy are created by modifying an HIV virus—"disarming" it—and then using it to change the DNA of patients' T cells, which are central to the human immune system. This synthetic biological engineering creates "chimeras" that are equipped with receptors on their surface (CARs) that enable the T cells to identify and attach themselves to a specific antigen (a protein) on cancer cells and kill them. Right now, CAR-T is the most advanced in successfully treating cancer patients, but other promising types of ACT therapies are also being developed. As we recounted, six-year-old Emily Whitehead, dying of acute lymphoblastic leukemia (ALL) in 2012, was the first child whose life was saved by CAR-T therapy.

This breakthrough in a pediatric clinical trial with a biotechnology, which took decades to develop, was just the beginning. Hundreds of children and young adults with ALL would be candidates for CAR-T to treat the most common cause of childhood cancer death, as would many adults who were dying of diffuse large B-cell lymphoma, the most common form of non-Hodgkin's lymphoma. In historic firsts for immunotherapy, the FDA approved CAR-T immunotherapies for both types of cancer in 2017. None of this would be possible without the human engineering of synthetic living molecules that are not available in nature. More breakthroughs like these undoubtedly are to come, even though no one can know precisely what and when.

CAR-T studies aimed at new drug targets for diseases like cancer will combine patient experiences, their medical records, genetics, and drug effects with artificial intelligence (AI). Although these studies are very high tech, they raise familiar bioethical issues about coercion and privacy, as in large-scale vaccination studies like those that helped establish polio vaccination policies in the 1950s. The benefits of a mass vaccination program must be overwhelming in order to justify the physical intrusion of an injection, a pill, or a liquid drink on people who are usually not ill, including children, sometimes without parental consent, as well as monitoring the movements of at-risk populations. Even if there is no direct physical contact with a number of individuals in a population—say, a sociological study of the way people swarm the shop doors at a New Year's Day sale—the privacy of those eager buyers as individuals must be respected. Data science should not repeat the errors of online marketing as when devices are inserted to track online buying habits or when massive quantities of information are gleaned from social media to guide advertising or to design ideological and political campaigns that manipulate public opinion. Preserving public trust in science requires a far higher level of respect for privacy than the worlds of commerce and politics.

But there's also a positive flip side to monitoring internet use that needs to be stressed because it can increase the predictive power of epidemiological studies and save lives. Google has claimed that, by tracking internet searches for flu-like symptoms, its search engine was able to anticipate the 2008 flu epidemic before the Centers for Disease Control and Prevention. The internet can also provide web searchers with up-to-date information about where to be vaccinated, much the way that advertisers work off of searches for relevant products. The social networks that are represented in online contacts might also aid in identifying people at risk for suicide. However, at the same time, social media may also stimulate and aggravate mental health problems, such as anxiety and eating disorders, especially in adolescents. Like most any technology, the internet has upsides and downsides. But its necessity and near omnipresence in everyday life makes our collectively coming to ethical terms with its use all the more important.

Although web searches are deliberate activities, the uses of those keystrokes by third parties are often beyond the control of the person using the search engine. Large quantities of possibly useful information can also be gleaned from aggregating many patients' clinical records: much information is created and summarized in the course of medical treatment on patient records that could be useful to learning about a disease beyond any particular patient.

Imagine, for example, that you have been diagnosed with a form of cancer and that there are a few different kinds of chemotherapy available. Like the vast majority of adults with cancer, instead of entering a clinical trial where your experience with a drug would be a matter of record and analyzed by experts, you and your local doctor settle on a particular approach for your disease. The chemotherapy you choose has been through rigorous clinical trials, but patients respond differently, especially in the real world outside an intensely monitored trial. At least one company has been formed to obtain all that patient experience and to develop software that can connect patients and their doctors to more effective and efficient treatments. This is a form of personalized medicine—the practice of tailoring treatments to individual patients.

For both practical and ethical reasons, these very promising and ingenious efforts must be made worthy of the public trust. Britain's Nuffield Council on Bioethics has been among the first bioethics groups in the world to ethically assess the new opportunities that information technology presents for large amounts of data. "How," they ask, "may we define a set of morally reasonable expectations about how data will be used in a data initiative, giving proper attention to the morally relevant interests at stake?" Their answer: privacy and clear disclosure of data use, individual freedom to modify consent forms, and ways to ensure that participants' reasonable expectations will be met are all critical.

Big data can come from small places. Related to the goal of personalizing medicine through clinical studies, a consumer industry has grown up around individualized genetic information or "personal genomics." These "spit-in-a-cup" commercial services offer to tell their customers about gene variants that could be related to our current or future health status or ancestry. There's a lot to be said for satisfying curiosity about the fruits of science, including that many of us might find the results of these direct-to-consumer (DTC) genetic tests personally compelling. Who wouldn't want to know what science can tell us about what diseases we might be prone to, or which ones we don't have to worry about, or who "my people" were ten generations ago?

DTC genetic testing drives science "home" in an accessible way that is unusual in these days of rarefied and highly specialized knowledge.

The practical and ethical importance of clearly informing DTC consumers of what they're getting—and not getting—by way of meaningful information cannot be exaggerated. Unlike finding new genetically appropriate treatments, as in CAR-T studies, the very meaning let alone usefulness of these tests for an individual's genetic fate typically isn't at all clear. Just as there is usually not a "gene for" a certain disease or quality, so too there is rarely a clear answer about genetic risks or benefits. When there is, as in the association of BRCA1 and BRCA2 genes with lethal forms of breast and ovarian cancer, women who are likely to benefit from being tested also need access to expert counseling about their results. To produce or to prevent a disease or a trait, most genes basically await a complex array of triggers (environment, diet, lifestyle, and luck), including interactions with some of our other twenty thousand genes, not to mention the DNA in our guts that isn't "us" (in any interesting social sense).

Today, the promise of preventing disease onset through a unique combination of measures learned by DTC testing is more hype and hope than heaven. Some customers don't know they can get bad news about which there's nothing to be done. This assumes the DTC tests are accurate. One careful study found that 40 percent of the results of raw data tests of genes from DTC companies were false positives. The FDA warned 23andMe in 2013 that inaccurate tests could pose a danger to customers. The company apologized and was later allowed to tell customers about some of their health risks such as for Parkinson's. An FDA officer noted, however, that "genetic risk is just one piece of the bigger puzzle, it does not mean they will or won't ultimately develop a disease."

The business model of this multi-billion-dollar industry also needs to be understood. DTC genetics companies could, if they chose, pay you to learn about your DNA and stockpile your genetic data along with that of other customers until it might be valuable, perhaps sooner than later. 23andMe is reported to have the largest biobank in the world and has moved into drug and disease research that draws upon such "big data." Because major benefits for patients come from the personalized medicine that depends on big data, we support efforts worthy of the public's trust to collect big data. Worthy efforts include making the public aware of risks to privacy. In 2018, 23andMe and a number of other genetics testing companies announced that they would ask for the customers' "separate express consent" before giving their genetic information to others, like drug companies doing medical research, and that information is "de-identified" so it isn't linked to individuals. But just a bit of digging into publicly available ancestry databases along with data from the Y chromosome can lead to the last name of a man in the United States. We agree with those who recommend placing a "caveat emptor!" ("let the buyer beware!") on the front page of every commercial website, with a clear statement that by providing your genetic information to these sites, you risk it being used for other, often unexpected, purposes.

Much social good can also come from unexpected uses of genetics, including in law enforcement. Few will object that the "privacy" of a vicious criminal was not respected in the course of solving a crime. Yet many were surprised when in 2018 a long-sought serial rapist and killer who had terrorized California residents was identified using publicly available big databases. He had gotten away for decades with killing over a dozen people and raping more than fifty women. How was the serial predator finally discovered? The captivating story featured the detective and DNA expert Paul Holes, with a hunch that he could find the criminal by obtaining a sample of his DNA and meticulously tracing his genetic ancestry by means of publicly available websites.

Detective Holes began by using the lesser-known, no frills GED-match. Using an alias, he submitted the killer's DNA sample from which he got his first set of clues, consisting of a few dozen distant relatives. Searching back to the early nineteenth century, he found a common ancestor they all shared and then used the well-known Ancestry.com to create family trees that he searched for suspects. The Golden State killer turned out to be a former police officer, which made him both less suspicious and more adept at eluding law enforcement. The outcome of this crime mystery underscored the distinctive power of DNA coupled with big databases to reveal identity. Since then, many other "cold cases" of murder have been reopened and the likely perpetrators identified using genetic databases. Legal challenges still await, but the various uses of DNA have already begun to transform the traditional concepts of what counts as personal and private information. GEDmatch not only told users that their site could be used for other purposes, but after discovering this unexpected use of their site, they posted a prominent warning that you should not upload your DNA or you should remove it if you don't want it used for other purposes, such as identifying your relatives who have committed crimes or were victims. This rapid response—prominently cautioning all users of potential uses of their genetic information—is a model worthy of emulation.

CRISPR

Sensitive to public and congressional concerns, when the Human Genome Project got started in 1990, it included a program on the ethical, legal, and social implications (ELSI) of genetic engineering. As expected, plenty of issues arose in short order. The ability to delete and replace segments of DNA got a rocket boost in the early 2010s when several American and European teams announced that separately they had developed a far more efficient technique than anything available to labs before—one that has come to be called gene editing. Within a few years, "crisper" was part of the popular science vocabulary.

CRISPR/Cas9 (CRISPR stands for "clustered regularly interspaced short palindromic repeats") exploits an ancient system that allows bacteria to acquire immunity from viruses. Unlike older bioengineering methods, CRISPR uses an enzyme or chemical catalyst to bind RNA to any DNA sequence chosen and to cut the DNA at that location, allowing researchers to insert new genetic material into the gap. Cas9 is the most popular enzyme used with CRISPR, whereas other enzymes are used for different experimental purposes.

Many diseases have been identified as potential targets for modifying genes in a patient's somatic or body cells, including sickle cell anemia, disorders linked to the maternal or X chromosome, hemophilia, cystic fibrosis, HIV/AIDS, certain forms of cancer, muscular dystrophy, Huntington's disease, and some neurodegenerative diseases. Developing therapies for these conditions using CRISPR will not be straightforward. Early laboratory work demonstrated, for example, that the human immune system may resist Cas9. Yet this needn't be a major setback since other enzymes are already being used for techniques associated with CRISPR. Using an older type of gene editing, a form of leukemia in infants has been successful as a bridge to transplanting bone marrow into a patient's body after the treatment, so the concept of gene editing for gene therapy has been proven. But significant obstacles need to be overcome in order to ensure safety, efficacy, and delivery to the many patients who can potentially benefit from gene therapy.

Along with the challenges of technical development, gene editing—like all the medically promising biotechnologies described in this chapter—raises a host of ethical issues, some familiar and some not. Although the idea of "unnatural" biological functions is alarming to some—apart from the concerns we discussed above about "playing God" and foolishly treating nature as a blank slate— the main issue is whether they are too risky or not. When it becomes scientifically feasible to try modifying body cells with gene editing in order to treat diseases, the same ethically sound rules that apply to any human experiment in gene therapy will apply to gene editing.

All research involving human gene editing in the United States, as we discussed in the journal *Foreign Affairs*, must meet the rigorous regulatory standards governing medical research. Some rules are formalized in regulation, as when scientists' work requires FDA approval or is supported by federal funds. Other rules governing human gene editing are informal, including self-regulation by the scientific community. The FDA advises researchers to follow up with participants in gene therapy trials for as long as fifteen years after the end of the trial to discover and deal with any delayed ill effects. And once the FDA approves gene therapy products for public sale, it requires companies to monitor their use, report any adverse events, and give public warnings as appropriate. This regulatory regime will be sufficient when it comes to using CRISPR to edit somatic cell genes given that the process, though different from other techniques of modifying cells, does not raise new safety or ethical issues.

The same cannot be said for modifications of an individual's germ cells, which carry genes that are inherited. Because they are inheritable, such germline modifications raise both the prospect of vast benefits and the most complicated questions of how to assess risks and benefits, not only in biological terms but also in global societal terms over the course of generations. It is no exaggeration to say that reengineering the human genome raises risks not only for individual patients but also for humanity as a whole. Unlike rapidly propagating species like mosquitoes, our human species is slow to reproduce in great numbers, so any biologically-damaging or societally-damaging change in a human germ line is likely to take decades or even centuries to become pronounced. All the more reason not to neglect these risks now. Adjusting one inheritable part of complex human biological systems could well have irreversible long-term consequences for public health and social well-being more generally.

The potential benefits of gene editing still must be considered alongside its risks. Gene editing could prevent the transmission of genes that increase the risks of life-threatening diseases, such as breast cancer or cystic fibrosis. Some families with histories of breast cancer associated with certain mutations in the BRCA1 and BRCA2 genes (which help prevent tumors), for example, may wish to protect their descendants by editing their genes. These modifications could take place in the setting of in vitro fertilization, with the select embryos then transferred to the mother for gestation. Survey results suggest that Americans largely agree with a 2017 National Academy of Sciences report that priority in gene editing research should be given to disease prevention rather than enhancement, even if that involves editing the germ line.

The prospects of disease prevention alone are far from enough to justify researchers taking it upon themselves to edit germ lines. This fact was dramatically driven home in 2018 when, without any apparent prior approval or notice, a team in China reported that they had genetically modified human embryos to resist a strain of HIV, resulting in the birth of twin girls. Their blatant failure to abide by many of the most basic ethical standards was met with appropriate outrage, sparking renewed pressure from the American and global scientific communities to make the rules and the sanctions against irresponsible gene editing more rigorous throughout the world.

Both the doing and the values of science require transparency. In the seventeenth century a group of brilliant natural philosophers like Robert Boyle and Christopher Wren thought of themselves as an "invisible college," exchanging ideas through the nascent postal system. In the twenty-first century, science communication is both instantaneous and global, creating a "global college" of scientists. But invisibility is no longer acceptable—or even possible for long. The funding and regulation of scientific work increasingly is and must be global. Countries and companies compete to originate and to market discoveries, but the ethics and benefits of biomedical science must not be treated as proprietary.

As technical proficiency in gene editing rapidly increases, many ethical issues will need to be addressed for true progress to be sustained: Is there clear disclosure of data use? Are there sufficient protections against the reengineering of heritable traits in ways that pose unmitigated risks to future generations? And will the benefits of new medical science be made available and affordable to those in need? When we can affirmatively answer these critical questions, we can also say that the future of opening cell doors is more hope than hype, even if not heaven. It holds out a realistic promise of contributing mightily to the constructive transformation of both public health and health care.

Epilogue

TRANSFORMING MINDS

Millions of years ago our ancestors could not avoid noticing how damaging a blow to the head could be. Nonetheless, human remains show that ancient surgeons were willing to cut holes in the skull, perhaps to relieve pressure, realizing that not all head injuries were the same. What made such injuries so different? Over the centuries the mysteries mounted. Working with a long iron rod topped with blasting powder, Phineas Gage, a nineteenth-century American railway worker, intended to poke a hole in some rock. Instead the powder picked up a spark and the rod pierced Gage's skull. Despite losing vision in one eye and much of the front of his brain, Gage survived. Though he was physically the same individual, many who knew him agreed that his personality was radically altered by the accident. He wasn't the industrious and responsible "old Phineas" anymore. Around the time of Gage's injury, the French surgeon Paul Broca found that when human patients lost an area in the front of the brain due to trauma, they also lost the ability to speak. Brain deficits have taught us a lot and not only from accidents. People born without a cerebellum, a large structure in the back of the brain, may be physically clumsy and forgetful but they still get on pretty well.

Today hundreds of thousands of veterans of wars in Iraq and Afghanistan suffer from traumatic brain injuries, as did veterans of almost all previous wars, following exposure to shock waves from improvised explosive devices or deployment-related accidents. The modern armor that protects the rest of their bodies does not fully protect their heads. Many veterans with traumatic brain injuries fail to respond to talk therapy or standard medications. Unlike Gage, their injuries are invisible, except when their tissues are put under a microscope, but are no less life changing. Millions of elderly people today live much longer owing to public health advances only to experience dementias like Alzheimer's. Among younger people, disorders like autism and psychotic disorders are also frustratingly resistant to medical progress.

Illnesses linked to the brain are among the most devastating and dispiriting sources of human suffering to patients, families, friends, and communities. Schizophrenia, typified by signs of psychosis, exemplifies the social impact of mental illness, the long struggle to improve treatments, and the dire need for advances in basic brain science. The antipsychotic medications of the 1950s and newer drugs have brought symptom relief for some, but they don't address the underlying disease nor adequately improve the ability to function in ordinary life. Holding a job, for instance, involves mental abilities that many people take for granted—like attention, concentration, and working memory—all disrupted by schizophrenia. At the moment, the prognosis for recovery is poor. Less than 20 percent of people with schizophrenia fully recover. For all the recent progress of neuroscience, scientific understanding of the most complex object in the known universe is not only an intellectual challenge, it is a moral responsibility.

ONE BRAIN, MANY PATHWAYS

Throughout *Everybody Wants to Go to Heaven, but Nobody Wants to Die* we have discussed many examples of the unavoidable moral choices that come along with medical progress. The challenges posed by these choices are individual, relating to hard decisions each of us must make for ourselves, our loved ones, and those who cannot speak for themselves, and they are also collectively challenging, as together we grapple with the roles of public and private institutions in advancing knowledge and providing health care. These are decisions that we cannot satisfactorily evade, though no hard decision will ever satisfy everyone.

The story of Parkinson's disease speaks to the urgency of pursuing better therapies for brain diseases and how different scientific strategies have contributed to progress so far. Animal research in the 1950s demonstrated that the amino acid L-dopa could reduce the distressing tremors associated with the disease. A few years later, brain autopsies of people with Parkinson's indicated lower than normal levels of the brain chemical dopamine. Doctors learned how to give patients L-dopa, a precursor to dopamine. The neurologist Oliver Sacks's book about L-dopa inspired a movie called *Awakenings*, which celebrated L-dopa therapy while also reminding audiences of its limitations and the sorrows associated with someone losing a sense of self. Decades later, advances in neuroscience contributed to the introduction of deep brain stimulation (DBS), an implanted device that sends electrical impulses to targeted groups of brain cells. DBS has also given many people back their lives, but it still only addresses the symptoms, not the underlying disease.

Drugs and devices can be greatly beneficial for all manner of illnesses and may work when nothing else does. But sometimes our bodies themselves can provide more basic and more straightforward resources for our well-being. For example, physical therapy can slow the progression of Parkinson's symptoms without the debilitating side effects of drugs or invasive surgery. Physical therapy's impact on the brain also teaches an important lesson here, one that has been suspected for well over a century and too often neglected to our detriment. The brain not only lies behind what we think and do but it is also changed, often profoundly, by what we think and do. A powerful feedback loop operates between the remarkable three-pound organ in our heads and the environment in which it has evolved, including the social environment we consciously provide it with our intentional actions. Among those actions, in addition to physical exercise and therapy, are meaningful work; intellectual, aesthetic, and athletic avocations; civic associations; friendships; and loving relationships. This list is far from exhaustive but it helps to convey the vast range of social activities we may decide to do in any given day that both emanate from and give feedback to our brains.

A classic example of a powerful pathway linking our brains and social networks, with transformative effects on our lives, is the neurochemical oxytocin, which is strongly associated with attachment to other people, between infants and caregivers as well as between lovers. Aptly for both pairs, oxytocin is sometimes called the "cuddle drug." Higher levels of oxytocin tend to mean less stress along with a sense of safety. Experiments indicate that when people are given a concentration of oxytocin through their nasal passages, they are more trusting. But we are not reducible to our brain chemistry any more than to our social relationships. Neuroscience demonstrates that our brain chemistry and social relationships have strong interactive effects that in turn influence our health and our life experiences. Taking a neuroscience course won't necessarily make someone more successful in manipulating oxytocin levels in their date's brain than anyone else. But neuroscience does offer major clues as to how we can better help ourselves and other people, including high-risk adolescents, to live healthier and longer lives, for example, by resisting the lure of tobacco and other harmful drugs, risky sexual behavior, drunken driving, and high-risk criminal behavior.

Government agencies have for decades mounted public health advertising campaigns to reduce smoking before it was prohibited in many public spaces and to increase the use of seat belts before they were commonly mandated. These campaigns often drew on behavioral science findings to hone their messages, the results leaving room for major improvement. In the case of seat belts, campaigns tried to get more passengers to buckle up with messages like "Make It Click—Buckle Up" and "It's a nice way to say I love you." Though some dispute whether such messages are persuasive or manipulative, there's no doubt that these failed in their goal of getting more people to buckle up (although they may have paved the way forward by increasing public support for the use of seat belts). In 1985 New York State ran a more successful kind of campaign, relying primarily neither on persuasion nor manipulation but coercion, broadcasting: "Wearing a seat belt is now the law in New York State."

The seat belt saga is relevant to an ongoing debate about the ethics of public health advertising campaigns. At the same time as buckling up was becoming law, bioethicist Ruth Faden was keenly questioning whether public health advertising campaigns are justified. Can we support effective antismoking campaigns if they don't persuade people through reason (aka respect for individual autonomy) but they primarily work by appealing to our fears and other emotions (aka manipulation)? Faden's way of answering this question faces up to the fact that we cannot maximize all that we value, either individually or collectively. We need to decide when appealing primarily to reason may rightly be overridden in light of other worthy considerations, such as saving lives, protecting nonsmokers, supporting a widespread agreement that these are worthy goals, and responding to unhealthy manipulations by commercial interests.

Neuroscience in this century has found even more effective messages that either short-circuit or preferably supplement our conscious reasoning and motivate us to choose healthier pathways. Neuroscientists now use brain imaging, often fMRI (functional magnetic resonance imaging) to track blood flow through different parts of each experimental subject's brain. They compare what subjects say will be most effective with the way their brains respond to different antismoking messages and images. Does the fMRI's "reading" of subjects' brains predict more or less accurately which message has the most power to promote public health compared with the message they actually tell the researchers will work best? Neuroscientists have demonstrated that *brains are often significantly better than conscious minds* at signaling what will most effectively motivate us to do the clearly healthier things that we should want to do. Still better predictions of public health campaigns have resulted from coupling brain imaging with self-reporting.

Some critics may consider any end run to our brains, around our conscious minds, an affront to autonomy. We consider it a happy irony: if autonomy is having good reasons for what we want to do, we can autonomously desire to be manipulated out of harmful addictive behaviors. In this limited sense, effective advertising campaigns that primarily appeal to people's emotions and aim at goals they consciously affirm can be reconciled with respect for individual autonomy. (There are other ways of using neuroscience findings, discussed below, that are far less friendly to autonomy or public health and safety.)

"MY BRAIN MADE ME DO IT"

Neuroscience is making great strides in helping us understand the underlying mechanisms that allow us to function as creatures endowed with minds and self-consciousness. Our minds emanate from our brains. But the progress of brain science itself is not what enables us to understand that we are morally responsible for our actions. A humanistic, ethical understanding recognizes our moral responsibility along with its limits when individuals are unable to comprehend what they are doing. Familiar human conditions that significantly limit moral responsibility or even eliminate it include infancy, when brains are immature, and serious brain injury. But under ordinary circumstances, no matter how much anyone insists that who we are is simply our brain, we still won't take "my brain made me do it" as an excuse for bad behavior.

Take, for instance, the mistaken conclusions that could be drawn from fMRI, which is probably the most impressive way to make images of brain activity. When computers with complex algorithms interpret brain data, they produce vivid images that purport to show where the brain "lights up" when the subject is engaged in a task like reading, watching a movie, or meditating. These images are based on correlations and are applied to an "average" brain, not the brain of the person who is actually being imaged. That doesn't make the images less impressive or less scientifically important, but we can't reasonably conclude that the images are "all there is" to reading, watching a movie, or meditating. It's not simply our brains that are doing these things—it is us. Our whole identity is not our brain.

The fMRI images of blood flow in the brains of people contemplating (or carrying out) crimes or considering (or telling) lies do not exempt those persons from accountability for their ultimate acts. And even if the brains of great scientists, writers, and humanitarians are "wired" differently from others, they are no less worthy of their Nobel Prizes awarded by virtue of their pathbreaking discoveries, novels, and contributions to world peace. We've also accepted some environmental explanations of crime and genius, as far as the facts can take us, without our needing to abandon the ethics and legality of holding people blameworthy and praiseworthy.

Because the brain is an electrochemical system, it can also be stimulated from the inside with electrodes to control tremors from diseases like Parkinson's or from the outside with electromagnetic pulses now being used to treat depression (as with DBS). In fact, our brains are modified all the time just by having ordinary experience, from the uterine environment to the qualities of the place where you are reading this page. That our brains change in light of their environment places special responsibility on those who aim to manipulate that environment.

Consider commercial advertising. Unlike our interactions with physicians and romantic partners, advertising appears to fall into that special kind of realm—along with political promises—where we expect to be misled but believe we can filter out the worst bits. Brain science provides tools that offer opportunities for manipulating behavior for reasons other than the improvement of mental or physical health. Nearly as soon as modern psychology became an established discipline, marketing executives saw its potential to sell products. In 1957 the journalist Vance Packard wrote a best seller called *The Hidden Persuaders*. Packard inveighed against "motivational research" that appealed to consumers' emotional needs and vulnerabilities rather than the quality of the item. To sell cake mix, for example, advertisers realized it was important to make the consumer feel like a real cook, so milk and eggs were added to the instructions on the box. Neither was necessary to make the cake.

Since the 1950s, brain science has built on motivational psychology with an array of devices. Electroencephalography (EEG), along with fMRI, has been applied to studies of the brain's response to commercials. For example, the stories presented in TV ads that activate brain areas associated with emotion tend to correlate with the person's brand preferences. That makes sense because we tend to remember events and what we read when an emotion is attached to them, a function performed by brain organs like the hippocampus. It's easy to see why companies eager to get an edge over the competition also hope that brain scanning can replace old-fashioned focus groups when they're considering a marketing campaign. At least one company claims that its headset can provide EEG measurements while people are shopping or watching TV ads.

This nascent field called neuromarketing also raises some novel and some familiar ethical questions. Is using a "mind-reading" gadget to sell products any more objectionable than asking a focus group to evaluate commercials or observing people in a store? Add to those individual and small-group responses all the "big data" that are available from the internet about the online behavior of masses of consumers. Facebook revealed in 2014 that it had deliberately manipulated the news feeds of nearly 700,000 users for one week to assess how negative and positive posts affected users' behavior. Here the territory of bioethics overlaps with that of business ethics and, what is more surprising, cybersecurity. Nobody knows at this point whether any company's or any country's hoped-for competitive advantage will devolve into a race in which no company or country has much of a lead for long.

What we do know is that the convergence of brain scans, big data, and the internet raises into high relief issues of privacy, the lack of either informed individual consent or democratic accountability, and the ability of powerful corporate actors to manipulate public preferences and behavior. Because our brains are networked into the physical and social environment, they can be powerfully manipulated by these techniques. Making use of behavioral data and the internet, social networking websites have created sophisticated algorithms that selectively "feed" us whatever they have calculated we most "crave" by messaging. When we react positively by responding to "clickbait," we contribute to their business model.

Using the tools of neuroscience to sell us stuff pales in comparison to those tools' potential for selling us ideas. At one level, brain technologies are hardly needed to do that. Influencing how we see the world has been accomplished and measured through data from the internet as it spreads through our social networks. Product marketers are learning about the effects of a brand name, logo, or video upon someone's brain as it's being scanned in a lab. They can then create a "neural profile" associated with responding to a certain brand. Companies can then profit from such brain scanning by selling their services to those intent on using this knowledge to disrupt a political system. By using the internet and social media, modern forms of marketing have become more efficient and correspondingly more dangerous.

Once false messages go viral, undoing the damage they've done becomes all but impossible. Governments intent on undermining their adversary's morale have long run propaganda campaigns that psychologically manipulate their target populations. Their approaches have ranged from Americans dropping leaflets on both civilian habitats and military targets to Japanese directing radio broadcasts at U.S. forces in the Pacific by female announcers whom the WWII troops famously called "Tokyo Rose." In the twenty-first century, nonstate actors are also prevalent, exploiting the internet and new social media instead of radio for political propaganda. Using these media with viral effects, the radical group ISIL (Islamic State of Iraq and the Levant) posted horrific videos of grisly beheadings beginning in 2014. Russian state-sponsored entities that have attempted to influence American elections since at least 2016 combine manipulative psychology, lies and deception, and social networks on the internet. Ironically, that internet was created by the Pentagon's cutting-edge science agency in the 1960s.

As public health campaigns that combat smoking and support healthy habits show, the news about marketing based on neural profiling isn't all bad, by any means. These tools have enormous potential—some of it already being realized—to improve human life by making the message of public health campaigns about harmful behaviors like substance abuse much more effective. The variety of applications of the new brain technologies is literally mind-boggling. An engaged public can guard against their dangerous uses, holding governments accountable, publicly criticizing companies and pressuring them into self-regulation, or calling upon governments to regulate and punish bad actors.

Regardless of what's going on in the neuroscience labs and how much researchers can learn from reading our brains, we still properly insist on holding individuals responsible for their actions under normal circumstances. In particular, our legal systems hold people legally accountable by implicitly distinguishing between what our brains do and what we can be held legally responsible for doing. Generally speaking, the standard of responsibility is the dominion of the law, not of neuroscience, while what our brains do is the dominion of neuroscience, not of the law. Short of external coercion or blackmail, like a threat against one's family, or preexisting evidence of insanity (mental disease that precludes awareness of one's actions, their meaning, or the ability to distinguish right from wrong), it is very difficult to exempt an individual from criminal responsibility in a determination of guilt or innocence.

In the absence of mandatory sentencing rules, courts may consider individual circumstances and states of mind in meting out specific individual punishments within a prescribed range. Extreme environmental deprivations and abuse, along with expressions of contrition, may similarly be factored into sentencing judgments (as long as such considerations are not ruled out by mandatory sentencing rules). These factors tend to be narrow and strict; they don't depend on brain scans and there's no reason they should. They typically reflect broad social judgments, which reach back millennia, about mitigating circumstances that may call for some degree of mercy.

Whether to be merciful, in what way, and to what degree are judgments that can't be determined solely on scientific grounds. To Mafia members who plead innocent because they were the victims of influence from bad people, our legal system says adults bear responsibility for the people with whom we associate. Meting out verdicts of guilt or innocence is consistent with a sound moral philosophy and legal system. Generally speaking, we can be held responsible and punished, even if in some technical sense "our brains made us do it."

BRAIN SCIENCE AND PERSONHOOD

Personal legal and moral responsibility is compatible with our modern understanding of the brain as closely tied to our personhood, so experiments with the human brain and its parts raise deep ethical issues. For example, the neuroscientist Irving Weissman was working in the early 2000s on the mechanisms of certain human brain diseases. Surgeons were already putting a relatively small number of human neural cells into animals to see whether they could "grow out" cancer cells. Weissman noted it was possible to go further, to make a mouse with a brain composed almost entirely of human brain cells from human stem cells. That human-mouse chimera (an animal with DNA from at least two different sources) would be a platform for studying the effects of drugs on diseases like Parkinson's. These experiments cannot be done with a human being.

Earlier we discussed the ethics of chimeric lab animals, creatures that have cells from different sources. Those animals don't in themselves create ethical issues. What's different about a mouse with only human brain cells instead of, say, a liver with all human liver cells? Modern humans consider the brain to be the seat of the self, of consciousness—not only cognition but also the entire range of human emotions—and much of what we both identify with and distinctively value about being a person. It matters a great deal if a mouse's behavior starts to resemble anything that we remotely associate with distinctively human behavior. From this disconcerting realization much provocative science fiction flows.

Suppose the behavior of the chimeric mouse (with human brain cells) wasn't different or the mouse didn't have some kind of "human thought" or "human self-consciousness." It still strikes many people that these kinds of experiments risk crossing lines between human and nonhuman beings, presenting dangers yet unknown and perhaps unknowable except in the long run when it might be too late to turn back. We sympathize with these concerns because we recognize the unique place of the brain in our self-understanding, but we also don't want to deny any medical benefits of these experiments to future generations. Recognizing all of this, Weissman consulted his Stanford University colleague, law professor Hank Greely, who along with others considered Weissman's proposed experiment. Greely's group concluded that "if the results indicate human brain structures or human behaviors, or even significant ambiguity, the experiments should be stopped and reconsidered in light of the new information. We did not have recommendations about what any such reconsideration should conclude; we did urge that it proceed with great care."

Experiments involving animals are closely monitored for just the sorts of unanticipated events that these Stanford ethicists and scientists considered. But the ethical issues about experiments with brain tissue are not limited to animal or human studies. Recent work shows that brain tissue can be grown from stem cells into tiny models of neural systems or "brain organoids." These miniature organs (about the size of a lentil) are not anything like a functioning human brain or its substantial parts, but they reproduce enough of its characteristics to pose great promise as platforms for laboratory experiments to understand the basics of brain diseases like schizophrenia that cannot be reproduced in animals. Because manipulating and growing human brain cells demands the most serious ethical attention, a group of ethicists and neuroscientists has recommended that an ethical framework be developed to guide work involving these neural tissues in a dish.

Surprisingly perhaps, work on AI poses a greater potential challenge to human intellectual capacity than putting human brain cells into nonhuman animals. Even higher primates have certain physiological characteristics that will always distinguish them from us, but non-biological systems are not constrained by the same rules of evolutionary biology. In 1996, many chess aficionados were amazed when the chess master Garry Kasparov fell to IBM's Deep Blue. Then in 2016, the ancient Asian game Go, with vastly greater tactical options and outcomes than chess, was conquered by a system called AlphaGo. Based on their understanding of how biological brains operate, neuroscientists today are supplying some of the essential tools that can be applied in "neural networks" to design ever more powerful and creative computers. Many think it's likely that AI will reach the outer limits of the imaginations of science fiction writers. Far fewer have come to terms with what the potential "creativity" of computers—their ability to destroy human privacy, for example—would mean for the fundamental ethics of everyday human life.

Worries about animals or machines overtaking humans are hardly new. In his 1970 best seller *Future Shock*, Alvin Toffler wrote that:

> There appears to be no reason, in principle, why we cannot go forward . . . to build humanoid machines capable of extremely varied behavior, capable even of "human" error and seemingly random choice—in short, to make them behaviorally indistinguishable from humans except by means of highly sophisticated or elaborate tests. At that point we shall face the novel sensation of trying to determine whether the smiling, assured humanoid behind the airline reservation counter is a pretty girl or a carefully wired robot.

Outdated as is his reference to "a pretty girl" or using a reservation counter to buy a plane ticket, more striking is Toffler's assumption that we will still be able to distinguish between humans and nonhumans with an elaborate enough test. Google Assistant and similar products are working toward thoroughly conversational systems complete with "uh's" and "um's." It also turns out that physical robots on assembly lines and those used as companions for people with dementia often work better when they are not humanoid in appearance. In both cases, though, the online virtual assistant and the factory robot benefit from a version of a human function that is also precious: memory.

LIVING MEMORIES

The idea of memory is far more complicated than we usually appreciate. So far, no information storage system has been able to use memory the way even more modest life forms than human beings can. For good reasons, then, memory has long fascinated philosophers and scientists. Plato thought that all learning is remembering information from some eternal reality. The eighteenth-century Scottish philosopher David Hume argued that a person is a collection of mental events, so we are in large part what we remember. These views are controversial but clearly most of us act as if our memories— operating in the background of our consciousness, often recalled and reassessed—are an essential part of our personal identities.

Yet the extreme amnesiac described by the neurologist Oliver Sacks in his book *Musicophilia* still seemed to have a sense of self, even though he could only retain new memories for a few minutes. Every time he saw his wife he was delighted, as though he hadn't seen her in years, though he knew that they were wed. In his moving memoir *In Search of Memory*, neuroscientist Eric Kandel recalls both his groundbreaking work on the science of memory, by studying neurons in simple marine animals like crayfish, and how he and his family were forced to emigrate from his native Austria to establish a new life in America. What a loss it would have been if Kandel had not been able to share his story. Kandel's memory has remained sharp for nine decades, but memory loss is a common and serious medical and emotional problem. Recent work by neuroscientists is building on the work of Kandel and others, developing technology that can help restore memory in people with diseases like epilepsy. The hope is that these promising early results can eventually be applied to people with Alzheimer's and other dementias.

Not all memories of course are pleasant. Beyond petty embarrassments many of us would prefer to forget, especially from high school, the elimination of emotional associations with painful life events for trauma victims would be a life-changing procedure. Some studies have suggested that drugs called beta-blockers, used to treat people with heart disease, can blunt the emotions associated with memories of events that could trigger post-traumatic stress disorders. Unfortunately, other studies have yielded disappointing results, suggesting that we are still far away from a full understanding of the nature of memory. Nonetheless, what if someday memories could be selectively edited, along the lines of the film *Eternal Sunshine of the Spotless Mind*? Experiments on brain cells that store memories suggest that developing drugs or devices that selectively eliminate specific memories may someday be possible.

The implications of new therapies that could blunt or erase memory are profound, and not only in a grand philosophical sense. For example, the legal system requires witnesses. Would important testimony be lost or compromised if a victim chose memory therapy? Would that even be permitted? Memories are not only "in our heads," registered in the cells of individual brains; memories are a shared resource. They are transmitted and embellished through myriad cultural media—from family stories to the arts and to religion, news, social media, and digitized data. Memories make us who we are, but they also make us more than ourselves.

What do we mean by this? Many of our most meaningful, indelible memories are those of loved ones, friends, acquaintances, and occasionally strangers who make a strong impression upon us. We absorb their perspectives and meld them with our own. Psychologists call this "perspective taking." In this ineluctably human way, other people's lives become ours as well as theirs. Memories become the fabric of our self-narratives; they are the stories that we transmit to future generations.

In fact, we can and do hear the dead in our memories. In the beginning of this book, we recalled Amy's mother, Bea, who insisted that the doctor ask Amy's grandmother Eva for her consent to surgery, and Jonathan's mother, Zerka, who was deprived of the information to which she was entitled after her arm was amputated. The experiences of Bea, Eva, and Zerka dealing with life-and-death situations became our memories as well as critical parts of our life experiences. We did not need to be genetically related to them for this to be true. In fact, Amy's mother lost her biological mother at birth and was adopted by Eva. Those memories helped to shape us and to motivate us to write *Everybody Wants to Go to Heaven, but Nobody Wants to Die*. "The life of the dead," Cicero said, "is placed in the memories of the living."

Allied with our memories, our hopes and aspirations for the future propel us forward. The progress of brain science holds out the realistic hope of better treating autism and psychotic disorders, preventing devastating forms of memory loss, determining how best to nudge ourselves to healthier habits, and creating better lives for our family, friends, and fellow human beings. Scientific progress also always tests our ethics, and learning more about our brains is no exception. Just as it's easy to want to go to heaven without dying, it's also easy to want everything that neuroscience has to offer without recognizing its limits.

Neuroscientists can now demonstrate how human brains react to the widest range of external stimuli. The smell of a Cinnabon sets off our brain's craving for sugar and fat. Poignant stories spread by the internet and social media about children who became autistic because they received an MMR vaccine stimulated many parents to resist having their children vaccinated, even though the causal claim came from publicly discredited, fraudulent research. The more that neuroscientists show us how our brains drive our behavior, the more important it becomes to consider who must be held morally and legally responsible for what behavior. Medical science has always needed ethics to partner with it to propel progress.

GOODNESS SEEKING JUSTICE

There is significant progress to celebrate and much more to strive for. In only one generation, remarkable advances in medical care, access to information about choices, and informed consent have served millions of Americans very well. Take the example of breast cancer, which will strike one out of every eight women. Or colon cancer: one in twenty-four women will be diagnosed with it. Those fortunate enough to have good health insurance and health care are likely to live long lives. One of those women is Eva Gossman, a revered (now retired) college dean who also taught practical ethics with Amy.

Born in 1930, Eva eluded the Nazis during World War II before emigrating with her family to the United States in 1948. A righteous Christian woman risked her own life and that of her ten-year-old daughter sheltering Eva and her family in her one-bedroom house in Nazi-occupied Slovakia, a story Eva recounts in her moving memoir, *Good Beyond Evil*. Now eighty-eight years old, Eva is a survivor in another sense: she has survived three different bouts of major cancers, including two of breast cancer and one of colon cancer. No stranger to suffering and anxiety, and a self-described pessimist, Eva has not only survived, she has thrived through unimaginable yet not uncommon health ordeals. On a wintry morning, when Amy asked Eva's permission to recount her story, she had just come in from her daily three-mile walk. It was with a friend who could not walk briskly, so Eva went out again for a faster walk later in the day. A prized mentor to young and old alike, Eva makes the most of every day of her long life. Her story exemplifies the major strength and major failing of American health care.

Over the past four decades, Eva's vibrant longevity has been made possible by many high-tech screenings, three surgeries (one radical mastectomy, one simple mastectomy, and colon surgery), genetic tests, several major new drug discoveries, and ongoing expert medical examinations, diagnoses, and treatments. In December of 1999, over twenty years after her two mastectomies, Eva was diagnosed again with breast cancer. (Her first breast cancer was detected on her birthday in December 1975.) She endured the standard of care chemotherapy treatments, but by 2002, diagnostic tests demonstrated a gradual rise in her tumor markers, suggesting another recurrence of cancer. Fortunately, pathbreaking medical research had recently led to the discovery and clinical care approval of Trastuzumab, marketed as Herceptin. Widely considered a "miracle drug," Herceptin is extremely expensive but found to be cost-effective: for many women whose tumors are determined by genetic testing to be HER2-positive, regular infusions with Herceptin can put their otherwise deadly breast cancer into remission.

Eva's experience with cancer treatment represents a major transformation from the "doctors know best" and "therapeutic privilege" norms that prevailed through the mid-twentieth century. The pace of innovative drug discovery since then has also been nothing short of transformative. Throughout the course of her many tests and treatments, Eva was clearly informed about her options and actively involved in consenting to treatments, some of which were judgment calls.

Just as Eva's story illustrates the revolution in technical medical capability and in informed consent, it also conveys, as Eva herself put it, that in American health care, "capability and distribution are not in synch." Over the years, Eva repeatedly expressed concern to Amy and others about her treatments' high cost to society, costs that she and her family could not have possibly afforded to pay. When her doctors advised her—out of an abundance of caution—to continue on the Herceptin for longer than there is clear clinical evidence of its efficacy, she consented for several years and then, in consultation with her oncologist, decided to stop the infusions. She has continued with diagnostic blood tests. Her breast cancer and her colon cancer (for which she received eight months of chemotherapy) remain in remission. Countless breakthroughs in lifesaving medicine coupled with major advances in ethical patient care make inspiring stories like Eva's not only possible but also quite common. Yet for everyone who cares about living a good life in solidarity with the millions of uninsured and underserved Americans, these breakthroughs stand in stark contrast to the persistent failure of American society to afford them and their families access to excellent health care and lifesaving medical breakthroughs.

A TRANSFORMATION IN PROGRESS

Bioethics has been part of a remarkable transformation in American health care, but that process is far from complete. As children, we observed the last vestiges of medical paternalism. Expectations about telling patients the truth, requiring informed consent, respecting patient autonomy, and protecting experimental subjects have been radically transformed over the past half century. Bioethicists have articulated, debated, and defended those changes. As scholars, teachers, observers, critics, and sometimes as activists, they have been part of the transformation of American health care. If bioethics had not existed in response to all those sudden changes in doctor-patient relations, it would have had to be invented.

The principle of respect for autonomy, doctors' duty to obtain informed consent, and other bioethical values have achieved an overwhelming measure of acceptance in American health care, but the same cannot be said about any principle of justice concerning providing health care to everyone. There are many reasons for this failure. Major divides over what constitutes justice are as old as philosophy itself. Formidable differences remain among influential theories of justice. The justice of American health care reaches far beyond medical matters to the very political and socioeconomic structure of our society. This fact makes accessible and affordable health care in the United States especially vulnerable to America's brand of partisan politics, short-term thinking, and powerful special interests. American government was designed to make it easier to block than to pass major national legislation, to protect citizens against overweening state power rather than to legislate for a controversial common good, even one with majority support. So for all the national political battles to extend affordable health care, going back almost a century, the United States remains the only major industrialized country—and the wealthiest one in the world—that has yet to provide it, or even to insure everyone for catastrophic illness.

Bioethics situates itself in response to different social and political systems. The American health care system is increasingly unaffordable, costing so much more than it does in any other country yet achieving so much less for the average American and especially for the most vulnerable. This inequity of our society's health care system has great potential to mobilize Americans for a common good. Our country's health care choices will reveal our priorities and challenge our determination to afford everybody the health care to which they are rightfully entitled. Both the transformation and the quest for justice in American health care are unfinished stories that continue to test the power of our compassion as well as our reason.

ACKNOWLEDGMENTS

No authors are islands. From across the world and over four decades, wonderful colleagues, students, and friends, too numerous to call out and thank by name here, have contributed to our understanding of these important bioethical issues.

Our experience with the Presidential Commission for the Study of Bioethical Issues informed our thinking on many matters. We are grateful to President Barack Obama for creating the commission, to Vice President Joe Biden, and Health and Human Services secretary Kathleen Sebelius for their support, and to Vice Chair Jim Wagner and our fellow commission members, executive directors, and staff for their multidisciplinary expertise and exemplary teamwork. Our thanks as well to Adam Michaels for providing expert staff support to Amy as chair of the commission, plus skillful referencing on the penultimate draft, faithful proofreading, and more.

We were also delighted to be able to recruit a previous commission staffer, Michael Tennison, as our meticulous fact checker and research assistant. Josh Green proofed the galleys. Any remaining errors are our own.

Greg Rost expertly managed all things logistical. Jodi Sarkisian, Mike Marco, and Michelle Jester handled countless details in the course of our collaboration.

A source of great encouragement, Eva Gossman generously allowed us to share her medical history along with her inspiring life story. Dorothy Roberts advised us on the history and legacy of race and

racial discrimination in medical science and practice. Abigail Erd-
mann suggested how best to present our personal stories in the Introduction and to express many complex issues throughout the book.
Marie Nicolini provided insight into euthanasia policies in Europe.
Tom Beauchamp enabled us to better understand the origins of some
key concepts in bioethics.

We are grateful to University of Pennsylvania (Penn) faculty, students, staff, trustees, and alumni for their support and inspired by the
multidisciplinary knowledge of health care, science, and technology
that they so generously share.

Amy thanks Dennis F. Thompson for coauthoring their work on
deliberative democracy and for their earlier co-teaching and writing
on ethics and public policy, experiences from which we have drawn.

Skip Gates first suggested to Amy that she might want to write a
book in his Norton series, an invitation she gratefully accepted before
her Penn presidency preempted her ability to write the book in time
for that series. Without that invitation, this book might never have
been written.

At Norton, Roby Harrington along with Robert Weil believed in
this project before we put any words on paper. Once we did, Weil's
editing proved invaluable. We thank them for their confidence and
expert guidance. Nina Hnatov copyedited with painstaking care.
With expertise matched by cheer, Gabriel Kachuck and Marie Panto-
jan guided the book to birth through its many stages of development.

Our loving thanks go to our spouses Michael Doyle and Leslye
Fenton who wisely advised on matters great and small, including
chapter titles and the subtleties of television medical shows.

NOTES

Introduction: A DUTY TO TELL

11 **achieving eternal perfection:** Year of origin unknown but first historical attribution is to Tom Delaney, an African American blues and jazz composer, in *The Afro-American*, October 16, 1948. Later also performed by country stars such as Loretta Lynn.

12 **The lives are identifiable:** Daniel Kahneman, *Thinking, Fast and Slow* (New York: Farrar, Straus and Giroux, 2011).

12 **a case of "lifeboat ethics":** Garrett Hardin, "Lifeboat Ethics: The Case Against Helping the Poor," *Psychology Today* (September 1974).

13 **How much health care spending:** Politifact, accessed September 14, 2018, https://www.politifact.com/truth-o-meter/statements/2013/oct/28/nick-gillespie/does-emergency-care-account-just-2-percent-all-hea/.

15 **the recent decrease in life expectancy in the United States:** Lenny Bernstein, "U.S. Life Expectancy Declines Again, A Dismal Trend Not Seen Since World War I," *Washington Post*, November 29, 2018, https://www.washingtonpost.com/national/health-science/us-life-expectancy-declines-again-a-dismal-trend-not-seen-since-world-war-i/2018/11/28/ae58bc8c-f28c-11e8-bc79-68604ed88993_story.html?utm_term=.7fcf78ee8356.

17 **textbook called *Medical Ethics*:** Edwin F. Healy, *Medical Ethics* (Chicago: Loyola University Press, 1956), 45.

19 **"Euphemisms are the general rule":** Donald Oken, "What to Tell Cancer Patients: A Study of Medical Attitudes," *JAMA* 175, no. 13 (1961): 1120–28.

20 **"the silent world of doctor and patient":** Jay Katz, *The Silent World of Doctor and Patient* (New York: Free Press, 1984), xiv.

21 **And "seeing" patients also competes:** Sciencedaily, accessed October 13, 2018, https://www.sciencedaily.com/releases/2014/01/140124115750.htm.

21 **ubiquitous screens in the modern consulting room:** Atul Gawande, "Why Doctors Hate Their Computers," *New Yorker*, November 12, 2018.

One: CHANGING TIMES

29 **"in the early 1960s":** Rosemary Stevens, "Health Care in the Early 1960s," *Health Care Financing Review* 18, no. 2 (1996): 11–22.

30 **"a stunning loss of confidence":** Paul Starr, *The Social Transformation of American Medicine: The Rise of a Sovereign Profession and the Making of a Vast Industry* (New York: Basic Books, 1982), 379.

30 **"We can expect additional pressure":** Rashi Fein, "Toward Adequate Health Care: Why We Need National Health Insurance," *Dissent* (Winter 1988), http://dissent.symionic.com/article/toward-adequate-health-care-why-we-need -national-health-insurance.

30 **trust in the medical profession:** Robert J. Blendon, John M. Benson, and Joachim O. Hero, "Public Trust in Physicians: U.S. Medicine in International Perspective," *New England Journal of Medicine* 371, no. 17 (October 2014): 1570–72.

30 *JAMA* **published a new survey:** Dennis Novack et al., "Changes in Physicians' Attitudes toward Telling the Cancer Patient," *JAMA* 241, no. 9 (March 1979): 897–900.

33 **appear on screen less often:** UCR, "Poor Ben Casey! Dr. Maggie's Switching Roles from That of Anesthesiologist," *Desert Sun* 36, no. 268 (June 14, 1963), 14.

34 **Falco won the Emmy:** Eric Deggans, "'Nurse Jackie' Ends as TV's Most Honest Depiction of Addiction," NPR, April 12, 2015, https://www.npr .org/2015/04/10/398713112/nurse-jackie-ends-as-tvs-most-honest-depiction-of -addiction.

35 **But bioethics today is different:** Healy, *Medical Ethics*, 45.

35 **When Katz described the traditional:** Katz, *Silent World*, xiv.

35 **"Every human being of adult years":** *Schloendorff v. Society of New York Hospital*, 211 N.Y. 125, 129–30, 105 N.E. 92, 93 (1914).

36 **In the courts 1972 was a pivotal year:** Ruth Faden and Tom L. Beauchamp, *A History and Theory of Informed Consent* (New York: Oxford University Press, 1986), 132–38.

36 **three legal cases:** For more on these legal developments *see* Faden and Tom Beauchamp, *A History and Theory of Informed Consent*, 32-34.

37 **a new professional organization:** Thomas K. McElhinney and Edmund D. Pellegrino, "The Institute on Human Values in Medicine: Its Role and Influence in the Conception and Evolution of Bioethics," *Theoretical Medicine and Bioethics* 22, no. 4 (August 2001): 291–317.

38 **Their foundation supported the production of the film:** Armand M. Antommaria, "'Who Should Survive? One of the Choices on Our Conscience': Mental Retardation and the History of Contemporary Bioethics," *Kennedy Institute of Ethics Journal* 16, no. 3 (September 2006): 205–24.

39 **that mouthful morphed into:** Albert R. Jonsen, *The Birth of Bioethics* (New York: Oxford University Press, 1998).

39 **A new journal:** "Front Matter," *Philosophy and Public Affairs* 1, no. 1 (Autumn 1971): 1–2.

40 **The philosopher and bioethicist Norman Daniels applied Rawls's prin-**

ciple: Norman Daniels, *Just Health Care* (Cambridge: Cambridge University Press, 1985).

40 **a distinctive "capability approach":** Amartya Sen, *Commodities and Capabilities* (New York: Oxford University Press, 1999).

40 **defended the most minimal state:** Robert Nozick, *Anarchy, State, and Utopia* (New York: Basic Books, 1974), 169, 235.

41 **universal health care is an "affordable dream":** Amartya Sen, "Universal Health Care: The Affordable Dream," *Harvard Public Health Review* 4 (2015), http://harvardpublichealthreview.org/universal-health-care-the-affordable-dream/.

41 **insurance-paying jobs or more money:** As discussed in Amy Gutmann, "For and Against Equal Access to Health Care," *Milbank Memorial Fund Quarterly* 59, no. 4 (1984): 542–60.

41 **Daniels argued strongly for affordable access:** Norman Daniels, "Equity of Access to Health Care: Some Conceptual and Ethical Issues" (paper delivered to the President's Commission for the Study of Ethical Issues in Medicine and Biomedical and Behavioral Research, Washington, DC, March 13, 1981).

42 **"be distinguished from the ethics of aiming at complete equality":** Sen, "Universal Health Care."

42 **The libertarianism of the economist and philosopher F. A. Hayek:** Friedrich A. Hayek, *The Road to Serfdom* (New York: Routledge, 1944), 125.

42 **Hayek denounced the "mirage of social justice":** Friedrich A. Hayek, *Law, Legislation and Liberty, Volume 2: The Mirage of Social Justice* (Chicago: University of Chicago Press, 1976).

43 ***Ought implies can:*** Immanuel Kant, *Critique of Pure Reason* (1781) (Cambridge: Cambridge University Press, 1999).

Two: BIOETHICS GOES PUBLIC

45 **"an established part of medical education":** Jonsen, *Birth of Bioethics*, 361.

46 **One congressional mandate to the National Commission:** Pub. L. No. 93-348 § 202(a)(1)(A), 88 Stat. 342, 349 (1974), https://www.gpo.gov/fdsys/pkg/STATUTE-88/pdf/STATUTE-88-Pg342.pdf.

46 **In its landmark *Belmont Report*:** The National Commission for the Protection of Human Subjects of Biomedical and Behavioral Research, *The Belmont Report: Ethics Principles and Guidelines for the Protection of Human Subjects of Research* (Washington, DC, 1979), https://www.hhs.gov/ohrp/regulations-and-policy/belmont-report/read-the-belmont-report/index.html.

46 **In their *Principles of Biomedical Ethics*:** Tom L. Beauchamp and James F. Childress, *Principles of Biomedical Ethics* (New York: Oxford University Press, 2012).

47 **short documentary made in the early 1970s:** *Please Let Me Die*, produced by Dax Cowart and Robert White (1974), DVD.

49 **A much longer documentary:** *Dax's Case*, produced by Unicorn Media, Inc. for Concern for Dying (1985), DVD.

50 **"protection of the confidential character":** *Tarasoff v. Regents of University of California*, 17 Cal. 3d 425, 442 (1976).

51 **A dissenting opinion:** Tarasoff (J. Clark, dissenting).

51 **"bad law, bad social science, and bad social policy":** Donald N. Bersoff, 2013 Presidential Address to the American Psychological Association, described in Donald N. Bersoff, "Protecting Victims of Violent Patients While Protecting Confidentiality," *American Psychologist* 69, no. 5 (2013): 461–67.

51 **While many U.S. states have since adopted:** Rebecca Johnson, Govind Persad, and Dominic Sisti, "The Tarasoff Rule: The Implications of Interstate Variation and Gaps in Professional Training," *Journal of the American Academy of Psychiatry and the Law Online* 42, no. 4 (2014): 469–77.

51 **A young Australian philosopher:** Peter Singer, *Animal Liberation* (New York: HarperCollins, 1975).

52 **Harking back to Bentham's famous (or infamous) position:** Jeremy Bentham, *Rights, Representation, and Reform: Nonsense upon Stilts and Other Writings on the French Revolution*, eds. Philip Schofield, Catherine Pease-Watkin, and Cyprian Blamires (New York: Oxford University Press, 2002), 330.

54 **A 1975 conference:** For example, *see* Paul Berg, "Asilomar 1975: DNA Modification Secured," *Nature* 455 (2008): 290–91.

56 **of such a clinically acceptable device (perfected or otherwise):** Shelley McKellar, *Artificial Hearts: The Allure and Ambivalence of a Controversial Medical Technology* (Baltimore: Johns Hopkins University Press, 2018), 25. Clark's suffering was not in vain. Although the goal of an artificial heart has not been achieved, this and other efforts have led to innovations like the left ventricular assist device (LVAD) that has extended many lives.

57 **Beginning in the late 1960s:** Jon F. Merz, Catherine A. Jackson, and Jacob Alex Klerman, "A Review of Abortion Policy: Legality, Medicaid Funding, and Parental Involvement, 1967–1994," *Women's Rights Law Report* 17, no. 1 (Winter 1995): 1–61.

58 **In 1969 an impoverished twenty-one-year-old:** *Roe v. Wade*, 410 U.S. 113, 164–65 (1973).

59 **Since 1973, the trends of American public opinion:** Gallup, "In Depth: Topics A to Z, Abortion," accessed September 14, 2018, http://news.gallup.com/poll/1576/abortion.aspx.

60 **The ethical core of the abortion controversy:** Amy Gutmann and Dennis F. Thompson, *Democracy and Disagreement* (Cambridge, MA: Belknap Press, 1998), 74.

60 **In his writing for the court:** *Roe*, 410 U.S. 113, 159.

60 **a "compelling interest":** *Roe*, 410 U.S. 113, 163–65. Before that point, as we noted, the court ruled that a woman's right to terminate her pregnancy must prevail, based on a right to privacy—with the proviso that state regulation is permitted between the first trimester and viability only in the interests of maternal health.

61 **philosopher Roger Wertheimer captured:** Roger Wertheimer, "Understanding the Abortion Argument," *Philosophy and Public Affairs* 1, no. 1 (1971): 67–95.

62 **Hastings Center cofounder Daniel Callahan and his wife:** Sidney Callahan and Daniel Callahan, eds., *Abortion: Understanding Differences* (New York: Springer, 1984).

63 **we can maximize that potential by economizing:** Gutmann and Thompson, *Democracy*, 85.

63 **in need of child support:** Amy Gutmann and Dennis F. Thompson, *Why Deliberative Democracy?* (Princeton, NJ: Princeton University Press, 2004): 89.

63 **Judith Jarvis Thomson creatively argued:** Judith Jarvis Thomson, "A Defense of Abortion," *Philosophy and Public Affairs* 1, no. 1 (1971): 47–66.

65 **Rather than subordinating the individual:** John Locke, *Two Treatises of Government* (1690), ed. Peter Laslett (Cambridge: Cambridge University Press, 1988).

65 **Immanuel Kant considered all persons:** Immanuel Kant, *Groundwork of the Metaphysics of Morals* (1785), eds. Mary Gregor and Jens Timmermann (Cambridge: Cambridge University Press, 2012).

Three: THE PUBLIC'S HEALTH

68 **Among preventative medical interventions:** John Halstead, "The Best Public Health Interventions of the 20th Century," *Giving What We Can*, April 25, 2015, https://www.givingwhatwecan.org/post/2015/04/best-public-health-interventions-20th-century/.

68 **By every standard measurement that is used:** Rebecca Masters et al., "Return on Investment of Public Health Interventions: A Systematic Review," *Journal of Epidemiology and Community Health* 71, no. 8 (August 2017): 827–34.

68 **High-technology medicine:** Aaron E. Carroll and Austin Frakt, "Save Lives. It Can Save Money. So Why Aren't We Spending More on Public Health?" *New York Times*, May 28, 2018; *see also* Muireann Quigley, "Nudging for Health: On Public Policy and Designing Choice Architecture," *Medical Law Review* 21, no. 4 (2013): 588–621.

68 **Tobacco control saved an estimated twenty-two million lives:** David T. Levy et al., "Seven Years of Progress in Tobacco Control: An Evaluation of the Effect of Nations Meeting the Highest Level MPOWER Measures between 2007 and 2014," *Tobacco Control* 27, no. 1 (2018): 50–57.

69 **The dramatic decline in childhood caries:** For example, *see* "Achievements in Public Health, 1900–1999: Fluoridation of Drinking Water to Prevent Dental Caries," *MMWR* 48, no. 41 (October 1999): 933–40, and Jane Brody, "25 Years of Fluoride Cuts Tooth Decay in Newburgh," *New York Times*, May 3, 1970, L64. Quote is from Dr. Maxwell Serman, in Brody, "25 Years of Fluoride," L64.

70 **deliberations about public health decisions:** Presidential Commission for the Study of Bioethical Issues, *Bioethics for Every Generation: Deliberation and Education in Health, Science and Technology* (Washington, DC, May 2016), https://bioethicsarchive.georgetown.edu/pcsbi/sites/default/files/PCSBI_Bioethics-Deliberation_0.pdf.

71 **As the public health scholar Nancy Kass:** Nancy Kass, "An Ethics Framework for Public Health," *American Journal of Public Health* 91, no. 11 (2001): 1776–82.

71 **Along with billions of dollars in other initiatives:** "Bill and Melinda Gates Give $4 Million for Malaria-Killing Mosquito: Here's How It Could Work," *Business Insider*, June 21, 2018, https://www.businessinsider.com/bill-gates -melinda-gates-malaria-killing-mosquito-2018-6.

72 **Andrew Wakefield, along with twelve coauthors:** Andrew J. Wakefield et al., "RETRACTED: Ileal-Lymphoid-Nodular Hyperplasia, Non-Specific Colitis, and Pervasive Developmental Disorder in Children," *Lancet* 351, no. 9103 (February 1998): 637–41.

72 **Brian Deer was able to uncover:** Brian Deer, "Andrew Wakefield: The Fraud Investigation," accessed September 14, 2018, https://briandeer.com/mmr/lancet -summary.htm.

73 **told in 2012 by Martine O'Callaghan:** Martine O'Callaghan, "Autism: A Mother's Story," *Vaccines Today*, June 22, 2012, https://www.vaccinestoday.eu/ stories/autism-a-mothers-story/.

74 **Nudging is a feature:** Richard H. Thaler and Cass R. Sunstein, *Nudge: Improving Decisions about Health, Wealth, and Happiness*, rev. ed. (New York: Penguin Books, 2009).

75 **Thaler has popularized the term "sludging":** Richard Thaler, "Nudge, Not Sludge," *Science* 361, no. 6401 (2018): 431.

75 **"It seems reasonable to say that people make good choices":** Thaler and Sunstein, *Nudge*, 9–10.

76 **One study found that people were most likely to exercise:** Neel P. Chokshi et al., "Loss-Framed Financial Incentives and Personalized Goal-Setting to Increase Physical Activity among Ischemic Heart Disease Patients Using Wearable Devices: The ACTIVE REWARD Randomized Trial," *Journal of the American Heart Association* 7, no. 12 (June 2018): e009173.

77 **Research findings are shedding more light on what works:** Jennifer L. Matjasko et al., "Applying Behavioral Economics to Public Health Policy: Illustrative Examples and Promising Directions," *American Journal of Preventive Medicine* 50, no. 5 Suppl 1 (May 2016): S13–19.

77 **Critics are concerned that its paternalism:** Jeremy Waldron, "It's All for Your Own Good," *New York Review of Books*, October 9, 2014.

78 **"Obesity and poverty," Bloomberg noted:** "Statement from Michael R. Bloomberg on Philadelphia's Tax on Sugar Sweetened Beverages," June 16, 2016, https://www.mikebloomberg.com/news/statement-from-michael-r-bloomberg -on-philadelphias-tax-on-sugar-sweetened-beverages/.

78 **The Pennsylvania Supreme Court upheld:** Laura McCrystal, "Pa. Supreme Court Upholds Philadelphia Soda Tax," July 18, 2018, http://www2.philly .com/philly/news/soda-tax-philadelphia-supreme-court-pennsylvania -20180718.html.

79 **Mental illness is the costliest condition:** Thomas Insel, "Post by Former NIMH Director Thomas Insel: Mental Health Awareness Month: By the Num-

bers," May 5, 2015, https://www.nimh.nih.gov/about/directors/thomas-insel/
blog/2015/mental-health-awareness-month-by-the-numbers.shtml.

79 **In the words of one historian of mental illness:** Andrew Scull, *Madness in
Civilization: A Cultural History of Insanity, from the Bible to Freud, from the
Madhouse to Modern Medicine*, Kindle ed. (Princeton, NJ: Princeton University
Press, 2015), 14.

79 **as many as half of all incarcerated individuals:** For example, *see* Olga
Khazan, "Most Prisoners Are Mentally Ill," *Atlantic*, April 7, 2015, https://
www.theatlantic.com/health/archive/2015/04/more-than-half-of-prisoners-are
-mentally-ill/389682/.

80 **Dominic Sisti has addressed a wide range:** Dominic A. Sisti, Andrea G. Segal,
and Ezekiel J. Emanuel, "Improving Long-Term Psychiatric Care: Bring Back
the Asylum," *JAMA* 313, no. 3 (2015): 243–44; Dominic A. Sisti, Elizabeth A.
Sinclair, and Steven S. Sharfstein, "Bedless Psychiatry: Rebuilding Behavioral
Health Service Capacity," *JAMA Psychiatry* 75, no. 5 (2018): 417–18; Andrea
G. Segal, Rosemary Frasso, and Dominic A. Sisti, "County Jail or Psychiatric
Hospital? Ethical Challenges in Correctional Mental Health Care," *Qualitative
Health Research* 28, no. 6 (2018): 963–76.

Four: UNEASY DEATHS

86 **Brittany Maynard, a twenty-nine-year-old:** Brittany Maynard, "My
Right to Death with Dignity at 29," CNN, November 2, 2014, http://www
.cnn.com/2014/10/07/opinion/maynard-assisted-suicide-cancer-dignity/
index.html.

89 **Simone de Beauvoir published a searing memoir:** Simone de Beauvoir, *A
Very Easy Death*, trans. Patrick O'Brian (New York: Pantheon Books, 1965).
Originally published as *Une mort très douce* (Paris: Gallimard, 1964). An experienced hospital social worker once observed that despite the good intentions
of dedicated professionals, "one person's personal emergency is another person's professional routine." That routine is transformed when physicians themselves are faced with serious illness. As oncologist Marc Garnick has written,
"until I became a patient, the accumulated burdens of treatment—the costs and
paperwork, challenges of dealing with specialty pharmacies, and the reactive
approaches to managing adverse events—that can sap a patient's will to perse-
vere had escaped my imagination. . . . Now when I say, 'I understand,' I really
mean it." Marc B. Garnick, "Filling in the Gaps," *JAMA* 319, no. 20 (May 22,
2018): 2079–80.

89 **moments of pointless torment:** de Beauvoir, *A Very Easy Death*, 81.

89 **a very easy death:** de Beauvoir, *A Very Easy Death*, 88.

90 **an upper-class death:** de Beauvoir, *A Very Easy Death*, 94–95.

91 **the American Heart Association recommended:** Mitchell T. Rabkin, Gerald
Gillerman, and Nancy R. Rice, "Orders Not to Resuscitate," *New England Journal of Medicine* 295 (August 1976): 364–66.

92 **heated courtroom drama:** For more on the "right to life" arguments, *see* Jill
   Lepore, "The Politics of Death," *New Yorker*, November 30, 2009, https://www
   .newyorker.com/magazine/2009/11/30/the-politics-of-death.

92 **The Quinlans lost that court case:** *In re Quinlan*, 70 N.J. 10, 355 A.2d 647
   (NJ 1976).

92 **Lewis Thomas coined the term:** Lewis Thomas, "The Technology of Medicine," *New England Journal of Medicine* 285 (1971): 1366–68.

93 **the publication of a presidential ethics commission's report:** President's
   Commission for the Study of Ethical Problems in Medicine and Biomedical
   and Behavioral Research, *Deciding to Forego Life-Sustaining Treatment* (Washington, DC: U.S. Government Printing Office, 1983).

94 **David Rothman observed in his aptly titled history:** David J. Rothman,
   *Strangers at the Bedside: A History of How Law and Bioethics Transformed Medi-
   cal Decision Making* (New York: Basic Books, 1991).

95 **In their influential textbook:** Beauchamp and Childress, *Biomedical Ethics*.

96 **two prominent critics:** Albert R. Jonsen and Stephen Toulmin, *The Abuse of Casuistry: A History of Moral Reasoning* (Berkeley: University of California Press, 1988).

96 **case analysis itself is incomplete without some guiding principles:** Jonsen
   and Toulmin, *Abuse of Casuistry*, 242.

97 **treatment would not be in his best interests:** *Superintendent of Belchertown
   State School v. Saikewicz*, 373 Mass. 728, 370 N.E.2d 417 (1977).

98 **"virtue is incomplete":** Richard B. Miller, *Casuistry and Modern Ethics: A Poetics of Practical Reasoning* (Chicago: University of Chicago Press, 1996), 17–18.

99 **an unsigned item entitled "It's Over, Debbie":** Name withheld by request,
   "It's Over, Debbie," *JAMA* 259, no. 2 (1988): 272.

100 **provoked vigorous protests:** Letters to the Editor, *JAMA* 259, no. 14 (1988):
    2094–95.

101 **this first unpleasant step can help establish:** Jack Kevorkian, *Prescription:
    Medicide: The Goodness of Planned Death* (Amherst, NY: Prometheus Books,
    1991), 214.

102 **that example was provided by Timothy Quill:** Timothy E. Quill, "Death and
    Dignity: A Case of Individualized Decision Making," *New England Journal of
    Medicine* 324 (1991): 691–94.

103 **As Quill wrote later:** Timothy E. Quill, *Death and Dignity: Making Choices
    and Taking Charge* (New York: W. W. Norton, 1994), 215.

104 **"civilization depends on the drawing of intelligent distinctions":** George F.
    Will, "Affirming a Right to Die with Dignity," *Washington Post*, August 25, 2015,
    https://www.washingtonpost.com/opinions/distinctions-in-end-of-life-decisions/
    2015/08/28/b34b8f6a-4ce7-11e5-902f-39e9219e574b_story.html.

104 **"the distinctive human dignity of autonomous choice":** Will, "Affirming a
    Right."

105 **they want access to physician-assisted death:** Timothy E. Quill, Robert M.
    Arnold, and Stuart J. Youngner, "Physician-Assisted Suicide: Finding a Path
    Forward in a Changing Legal Environment," *Annals of Internal Medicine* 167,
    no. 8 (October 2017): 597–98.

106 **By making the conditions of legalization stringent and specific:** Surveys reveal that about two-thirds of Americans support physician-assisted death. Surveys are notoriously susceptible to varying results (so-called framing effects) with different wording. Yet even when called "physician-assisted suicide," a majority supports the practice. *See* Ezekiel J. Emanuel et al., "Attitudes and Practices of Euthanasia and Physician-Assisted Suicide in the United States, Canada, and Europe," *JAMA* 316, no.1 (July 2016): 79–90.

107 **about the situation in various countries:** Emanuel et al., *Attitudes and Practices*, 79–90.

109 **Daniel Sulmasy calls it "intrinsic dignity":** Daniel Sulmasy, "Chapter 18: Dignity and Bioethics: History, Theory, and Selected Applications," in *Human Dignity and Bioethics: Essays Commissioned by the President's Council on Bioethics* (Washington, DC, March 2008), https://bioethicsarchive.georgetown.edu/pcbe/reports/human_dignity/chapter18.html.

109 **Sulmasy also interprets autonomy:** Jo Cavallo, "Debate over Legalizing Physician-Assisted Death for the Terminally Ill," *ASCO Post*, December 15, 2014, http://www.ascopost.com/issues/december-15-2014/debate-over-legalizing-physician-assisted-death-for-the-terminally-ill/.

109 **What's morally prohibited, they argue:** Daniel P. Sulmasy and Edmund D. Pellegrino, "The Rule of Double Effect: Clearing Up the Double Talk," *Archives of Internal Medicine* 159, no. 6 (March 1999): 545–50.

110 **This concept of human dignity:** For a fuller understanding of the concept of dignity as thoughtful self-determination, its historical roots, and its implications for public life, *see* George Kateb, *Human Dignity* (Cambridge, MA: Harvard University Press, 2011).

111 **the best available data from the United States:** Emanuel et al., *Attitudes and Practices*, 79–90.

111 **Ruth Macklin has argued that dignity:** Ruth Macklin, "Dignity Is a Useless Concept: It Means No More Than Respect for Persons or Their Autonomy," *British Medical Journal* 327, no. 7429 (December 2003): 1419–20.

112 **international human rights documents:** Universal Declaration of Human Rights, accessed September 14, 2018, http://www.un.org/en/universal-declaration-human-rights/.

112 **Central and Eastern Europe have been described:** Emanuel et al., *Attitudes and Practices*, 79–90

113 **"an intrinsic element of our humanity":** Daniel P. Sulmasy, "Health Care Justice and Hospice Care," special supplement, *Hastings Center Report* 33, no. 2 (2003): S14–15, https://www.growthhouse.org/nhwg/sulmasy_supplement.htm.

113 **This is a crucial first step:** This is an example of how people can economize on their disagreements by finding common ground amid ongoing deep disagreement. It's what Gutmann and Thompson more generally call the practice of economizing on disagreement (in *Democracy and Disagreement*). The October 17, 2017, issue of *Annals of Internal Medicine* (vol. 167, no. 8), for example, featured an editorial position against physician-assisted death, articles for and against, and a factual summary of the experience in Oregon. The articles

include "Oregon's Death with Dignity Act: 20 Years of Experience to Inform
the Debate," "The Slippery Slope of Legalization of Physician-Assisted Suicide,"
"Physician-Assisted Suicide: Finding a Path Forward in a Changing Legal Environment," and "Ethics and the Legalization of Physician-Assisted Suicide: An
American College of Physicians Position Paper."

114 **Yet for all this progress:** Paula Span, "A Quiet End to the 'Death Panels'
Debate," *New York Times,* November 24, 2015, https://www.nytimes.com/2015
/11/24/health/end-of-death-panels-myth-brings-new-end-of-life-challenges
.html.

114 **The baseless claim by former Alaska governor:** Robert Pear, "New Medicare
Rule Authorizes 'End-of-Life Consultations,'" *New York Times*, October 31,
2015, https://www.nytimes.com/2015/10/31/us/new-medicare-rule-authorizes
-end-of-life-consultations.html.

Five: THE HIGH PRICE OF UNFAIR HEALTH CARE

116 **The unfavorable trend has persisted:** Samuel L. Dickman et al., "Health
Spending for Low-, Middle-, and High-Income Americans, 1963–2012,"
Health Affairs 35, no. 7 (July 2016): 1189–96.

116 **rising by 20 percent:** Lenny Bernstein, "U.S. Life Expectancy Declines for
the First Time since 1993," *Washington Post*, December 8, 2016, https://www
.washingtonpost.com/national/health-science/us-life-expectancy-declines
-for-the-first-time-since-1993/2016/12/07/7dcdc7b4-bc93-11e6-91ee-1adddfe
36cbe_story.html?utm_term=.181fa1dc4e55.

116 **Anne Case and Angus Deaton had warned for years:** Anne Case and Angus
Deaton, "Rising Morbidity and Mortality in Midlife among White Non-
Hispanic Americans in the 21st Century," *PNAS* 112, no. 49 (December 2015):
15078–83.

116 **By 2015, for the first time on record:** "The American Middle Class Is Losing
Ground," Pew Research Center (December 2015).

117 **Rawlsian perspective developed by Norman Daniels:** John Rawls, *A Theory
of Justice: Revised Edition* (Cambridge: Belknap Press, 1999), 73–78, 263–67;
Daniels, *Just Health Care,* 36–58.

117 **Sen's "capabilities" perspective:** Sen, *Commodities and Capabilities.*

118 **By liberal lights, health care is a basic human right:** For a comparison to
other Western nations, *see* Commonwealth Fund, "New 11-Country Study:
U.S. Health Care System Has Widest Gap between People with Higher and
Lower Incomes" (July 2017); *see also* Sen, "Universal Health Care."

118 **Nozick opposed governmental redistribution for the sake of health care:**
Nozick, *Anarchy, State,* 169.

118 **Hayek vehemently rejected:** Hayek, *Road to Serfdom,* 37.

119 **"a comprehensive system of social insurance":** Hayek, *Road to Serfdom,* 125.

122 **millions of Americans read the remarkable story:** Shana Alexander, "They
Decide Who Lives, Who Dies," *Life,* November 9, 1962, 102–25.

123 **"worth" saving and whose death the least "costly":** Alexander, "They Decide Who Lives," 125.

123 **"a candidate who plans to come before this committee":** Alexander, "They Decide Who Lives," 118.

124 **"I frankly don't know":** Alexander, "They Decide Who Lives," 118.

124 **debated the amendment for thirty minutes:** Richard A. Rettig, "Origins of the Medicare Kidney Disease Entitlement: The Social Security Amendments of 1972," in *Biomedical Politics*, ed. Kathi E. Hanna (Washington, DC: National Academy Press, 1991).

125 **He was featured in an NBC TV documentary:** Richard A. Rettig, "The Policy Debate on End-Stage Renal Disease," *Law and Contemporary Problems* 40 (1976), reprinted in *Ethics and Politics: Cases and Comments*, 1st ed., eds. Amy Gutmann and Dennis F. Thompson (Chicago: Nelson-Hall, 1984).

126 **Gina Kolata reported:** Gina B. Kolata, "Dialysis after Nearly a Decade," *Science* 208, no. 4443 (May 1980): 473–76.

126 **some insurance companies are refusing to pay:** Katie Thomas, "Insurers Battle Families over Costly Drug for Fatal Disease," *New York Times*, June 22, 2017, https://www.nytimes.com/2017/06/22/health/duchenne-muscular-dystrophy -drug-exondys-51.html.

127 **The truth is, nearly every society:** Sen, "Universal Health Care."

127 **a presidential bioethics commission concluded:** President's Commission for the Study of Ethical Problems in Medicine and Biomedical and Behavioral Research, *Securing Access to Health Care* (Washington, DC: U.S. Government Printing Office, 1983).

128 **As dissenting Utah senator Wallace Bennett:** Rettig, "Policy Debate," 225.

128 **In reply to Bennett:** Rettig, "Policy Debate," 225.

129 **Deliberative democracy calls upon citizens:** Gutmann and Thompson, *Democracy and Disagreement*; *see also* the wide range of perspectives and practical applications of deliberative democracy compiled in André Bächtiger, John S. Dryzek, Jane Mansbridge, and Mark E. Warren, *The Oxford Handbook of Deliberative Democracy* (Oxford: Oxford University Press, 2018).

129 **"an essential response to authoritarian populism and post-truth politics":** Bächtiger et al., *Oxford Handbook*, 2.

129 **While no policy-making process is perfect:** Gutmann and Thompson, *Democracy and Disagreement*.

130 **"The absence of legislative hearings":** Rettig, "Policy Debate."

130 **philosopher and parliamentarian Edmund Burke:** For a deep understanding of Burke's life and philosophy, *see* David Bromwich's magisterial *The Intellectual Life of Edmund Burke: From the Sublime and the Beautiful to American Independence* (Cambridge, MA: Belknap Press, 2014); Michael Oakeshott (1991), "Rationalism in Politics and Other Essays," new and expanded ed., ed. T. Fuller (Indianapolis: Liberty Fund, 1991). Original edition London: Methuen, 1962.

130 **Burke was critical of the French Revolution:** Edmund Burke, *Reflections on the Revolution in France* (London: Dodsley in Pall Mall, 1790); for Burke's

view on the American Revolution, *see* http://www.oxfordscholarlyeditions.com/
view/10.1093/actrade/9780199665198.book.1/actrade-9780199665198-div1
-38?r-1=1.000&wm-1=1&t-1=contents-tab&p1-1=1&w1-1=1.000&p2-1=1&w2
-1=0.400#page329.

131 **David Brooks says in homage to Burke:** David Brooks and Gail Collins, "The Conversation: What Would Edmund Burke Say?," *New York Times*, October 21, 2014, https://opinionator.blogs.nytimes.com/2014/10/21/what-would-edmund -burke-say/.

132 **social historian Max Weber noted:** Quoted in Terry Maley, *Democracy & the Political in Max Weber's Thought* (Toronto: University of Toronto Press, 2011).

132 **described as "junk insurance":** Robert Pear, "'Short Term' Health Insurance? Up to 3 Years under New Trump Policy," *New York Times*, August 1, 2018, https://www.nytimes.com/2018/08/01/us/politics/trump-short-term-health -insurance.html.

133 **The AMA vehemently opposed:** Starr, *Social Transformation*.

134 **As Paul Starr's social history:** Starr, *Social Transformation*.

135 **Surveys indicate that 85 percent of seniors:** Meghan McCarthy, "Seniors Love Their Medicare (Advantage)," *Morning Consult*, March 30, 2015, https:// morningconsult.com/2015/03/30/seniors-love-their-medicare-advantage/.

137 **a complementary kind of conservatism:** Kahneman, *Thinking, Fast and Slow*, 283–86.

138 **60 percent of Americans say:** "Public Support for 'Single Payer' Health Coverage Grows, Driven by Democrats," Pew Research Center (July 2017).

139 **"a public relations disaster":** Paul Safier, "Rationing the Public: The Oregon Health Plan" in *Ethics and Politics: Cases and Comments*, 4th ed., eds. Amy Gutmann and Dennis F. Thompson (Belmont, CA: Thomson/Wadsworth, 2006).

141 **As far as outcomes, in extending health insurance:** Charles J. Courtemanche and Daniel Zapata, "Does Universal Coverage Improve Health? The Massachusetts Experience" (NBER working paper no. 17893, Cambridge, MA: National Bureau of Economic Research, 2014), https://www.nber.org/papers/w17893.

141 **After its major provisions went into effect:** Susan L. Hayes, "What's at Stake: State's Progress on Health Coverage and Access to Care, 2013–2016," Commonwealth Fund, December 14, 2017, https://www.commonwealthfund.org/ publications/issue-briefs/2017/dec/whats-stake-states-progress-health-coverage -and-access-care-2013#/.

142 **An important lesson of Romneycare:** For example, *see* David Cutler and Steven M. Walsh, "The Massachusetts Target on Medical Spending Growth," NEJM Catalyst, May 11, 2016, https://catalyst.nejm.org/massachusetts-target -medical-spending-growth/.

143 **"State officials, health care providers and local advocacy groups":** Margot Sanger-Katz and Quoctrung Bui, "The Impact of Obamacare in Four Maps," *New York Times*, October 31, 2016, https://www.nytimes.com/interac tive/2016/10/31/upshot/up-uninsured-2016.html.

145 **There are many ethically challenging issues in health care:** Elizabeth Rosenthal, "Nine Rights Every Patient Should Demand," *New York Times*, April 27, 2018,

https://www.nytimes.com/2018/04/27/opinion/sunday/patients-rights-hospitals
-health-care.html.

146 **suggested by the surgeon-scholar Atul Gawande:** Atul Gawande, "The Cost Conundrum," *New Yorker*, June 1, 2009; *see also* Atul Gawande, "Overkill," *New Yorker*, May 11, 2015.

147 **As several experts on the U.S. system point out:** Thomas J. Bollyky, Aaron S. Kesselheim, and Joshua M. Sharfstein, "What Trump Should Actually Do about the High Cost of Drugs," *New York Times*, May 14, 2018, https://www .nytimes.com/2018/05/14/opinion/trump-costs-drugs-pricing.html.

147 **The differences are glaring:** Irene Papanicolas, Liana R. Woskie, and Ashish K. Jha, "Health Care Spending in the United States and Other High-Income Countries," *JAMA* 319, no. 10 (March 2018): 1024–39.

147 **These differences are driven primarily by price:** Gerard Anderson et al., "It's the Prices, Stupid: Why the United States Is So Different from Other Countries," *Health Affairs* 22, no. 3 (May–June 2003): 89–105. Drug ads on television that include monthly prices are one way to call attention to the problem and perhaps, in the long run, cause consumers to put pressure on policy makers. But owing to the imperfections of the pharmaceutical marketplace and the fact that consumers are not usually the purchasers, price transparency is not the ultimate solution.

148 **Ezekiel Emanuel and others have pointed out:** Ezekiel J. Emanuel, "The Real Cost of the US Health Care System," *JAMA* 319, no. 10 (2018): 983–85.

148 **A major reason is that the United States spends less:** Austin Frakt, "Medical Mystery: Something Happened to U.S. Health Spending after 1980," *New York Times*, May 14, 2018, https://www.nytimes.com/2018/05/14/upshot/medical -mystery-health-spending-1980.html.

Six: FORAGING FOR ETHICS

153 **Kenneth Arrow originally observed:** Kenneth J. Arrow, "Uncertainty and the Welfare Economics of Medical Care," *American Economic Review* 53, no. 5 (1963): 941–73.

154 **Congress also should take steps to control exorbitant drug pricing:** Henry Waxman, et al., "Getting to the Root of High Prescription Drug Prices: Drivers and Potential Solutions," *CommonwealthFund.org*, July 10, 2017, https://www .commonwealthfund.org/publications/fund-reports/2017/jul/getting-root-high -prescription-drug-prices-drivers-and-potential. *See also* Daniel J. Kevles, "Why Is Medicine So Expensive," *New York Review of Books*, February 21, 2019, https://www.nybooks.com/articles/2019/02/21/why-is-medicine-so-expensive/.

155 **"one of the world's most pressing public health problems":** Centers for Disease Control, "National Antimicrobial Resistance Monitoring System for Enteric Bacteria (NARMS)," accessed September 14, 2018, https://www.cdc .gov/narms/faq.html.

156 **pictures of babies:** *See Life* magazine, August 10, 1962.

157 **"a fussy, stubborn, unreasonable bureaucrat":** Robert D. McFadden, "Frances Oldham Kelsey, Who Saved U.S. Babies from Thalidomide, Dies at 101," *New York Times*, August 7, 2015, https://www.nytimes.com/2015/08/08/science/frances-oldham-kelsey-fda-doctor-who-exposed-danger-of-thalidomide-dies-at-101.html.

157 **not only the toxicity:** Frances O. Kelsey, "Thalidomide Update: Regulatory Aspects," *Teratology* 38, no. 3 (1988): 221–26; *see also* FDA, "Kefauver-Harris Amendments Revolutionized Drug Development," accessed September 14, 2018, https://www.fda.gov/ForConsumers/ConsumerUpdates/ucm322856.htm.

158 **"more than 30,000 women":** Daniel F. Hayes, review of *False Hope: Bone Marrow Transplantation for Breast Cancer,* by Richard A. Rettig et al., *New England Journal of Medicine* 357 (September 2007): 1059–60.

158 **Yet in 2018 the Trump administration:** Editorial, "Want Reliable Medical Information? The Trump Administration Doesn't," *New York Times,* July 19, 2018, https://www.nytimes.com/2018/07/19/opinion/trump-medicine-data-hhs-ahrq.html.

158 **Inefficiency and unfairness are the mildest possible terms:** Editorial, "Reliable Medical Information."

159 **the 1990s was a "parallel track":** "Expanding Access to Investigational Therapies for HIV Infection and AIDS," Institute of Medicine Conference Summary (1991).

160 **the FDA responded with alternative pathways for access:** "Expanding Access."

160 **As painful and fitful as the process has been:** There is another dark aspect to the thalidomide story that was largely unknown at the time. The German company that developed it and attempted to cover up its harmful effects, Grünenthal, was then a safe haven for former Nazi doctors who were involved in murderous "euthanasia" programs and human experiments. One of the company's advisors was Otto Ambros, codeveloper of the nerve gas sarin. Ambros had been convicted at a Nuremberg, Germany, war crimes trial of using slave labor at the I. G. Farben chemical plant. Unfortunately, American companies can't claim clean hands as both Dow and W. R. Grace also employed Ambros, as did the U.S. Army Chemical Corps. The Grünenthal story is a disheartening reminder of the way that an individual's usefulness in business and national security can overcome even a record of barbaric cruelty. *See Newsweek,* "The Nazis and Thalidomide: The Worst Drug Scandal of All Time," September 10, 2012, https://www.newsweek.com/nazis-and-thalidomide-worst-drug-scandal-all-time-64655.

160 **libertarian party platform:** Libertarian Party, 2018 Platform, accessed September 14, 2018, https://www.lp.org/platform/.

161 **oversaw a monopoly:** John Hudak and Grace Wallack, "Ending the U.S. Government's War on Medical Marijuana Research," Center for Effective Governance at Brookings, June 2016, https://www.brookings.edu/wp-content/uploads/2016/06/Ending-the-US-governments-war-on-medical-marijuana-research.pdf; *see also* David Downs, "The Science behind the DEA's Long War on

Marijuana," *Scientific American*, April 19, 2016, https://www.scientificamerican
.com/article/the-science-behind-the-dea-s-long-war-on-marijuana/.

162 **DEA has no timeline for acting:** Hatch, Harris Call on Sessions, DOJ to Stop
Blocking Medical Marijuana Research, April 12, 2018, https://www.hatch
.senate.gov/public/index.cfm/2018/4/hatch-harris-call-on-sessions-doj-to-stop
-blocking-medical-marijuana-research.

162 **"conclusive or substantial evidence":** National Academies of Sciences, Engi-
neering, and Medicine, *The Health Effects of Cannabis and Cannabinoids: The
Current State of Evidence and Recommendations for Research* (Washington, DC:
National Academies Press, 2017), 127–28.

164 **As to the ethics of the operation:** "Heart Surgeon Christiaan Barnard Dies,"
Washington Post, September 3, 2001, https://www.washingtonpost.com/archive/
local/2001/09/03/heart-surgeon-christiaan-barnard-dies/82ab4aae-4854-462e
-96b3-dbf042ecadf4/.

164 **"A determination of death":** Uniform Determination of Death Act, 1980,
http://www.uniformlaws.org/shared/docs/determination%20of%20death/
udda80.pdf.

165 **the committee also intended:** "A Definition of Irreversible Coma: Report of
the Ad Hoc Committee of the Harvard Medical School to Examine the Definition of Brain Death," *JAMA* 205, no. 6 (1968): 337–40.

166 **"The Powerful Placebo":** Henry K. Beecher, "The Powerful Placebo," *JAMA*
159, no. 17 (1955): 1602–6.

166 **Despite predictions:** Rachel Aviv, "What Does It Mean to Die?," *New Yorker*,
February 5, 2018, https://www.newyorker.com/magazine/2018/02/05/what
-does-it-mean-to-die.

167 **They range from less controversial ideas:** James F. Childress and Cathryn T.
Liverman, eds., "Organ Donation—Opportunities for Action: Committee on
Increasing Rates of Organ Donation, Board on Health Sciences Policy" (Wash-
ington, DC: National Academies Press, 2006).

168 **like the bioethicist Arthur Caplan:** Arthur Caplan, "Bioethics of Organ
Transplantation," *Cold Spring Harbor Perspectives in Medicine* 4, no. 3 (March
2014), a015685.

168 **Spain—a Catholic country—had the highest rate:** International Registry in
Organ Donation and Transplantation, "Final Numbers 2016," December 2017,
http://www.irodat.org/img/database/pdf/IRODaT%20newletter%20Final%20
2016.pdf.

170 **distinguished by political philosopher Michael Sandel:** Michael Sandel,
What Money Can't Buy: The Moral Limits of Markets (New York: Farrar, Straus,
and Giroux, 2013), 93–130.

171 **"as a collection of spare parts":** Sandel, *What Money Can't Buy*, 110.

172 **prohibits donors from selling organs:** Julia D. Mahoney, "Altruism, Markets,
and Organ Procurement," *Law and Contemporary Problems* 72 (2009): 17–36.

172 **savings would include the costs:** Alexander M. Capron and Francis L. Delmonico, "Cover the Costs for Kidney Donors to Increase the Supply," *New York
Times*, August 22, 2014, https://www.nytimes.com/roomfordebate/2014/08/21/

how-much-for-a-kidney/cover-the-costs-for-kidney-donors-to-increase-the
-supply.

173 **we could greatly benefit low-income individuals:** For a thorough discussion
of organ markets, *see New York Times*, August 8, 2014, https://www.nytimes
.com/roomfordebate/2014/08/21/how-much-for-a-kidney.

173 **solid organs were transplanted:** Organ Donation and Transplantation
Activities, 2015 Report, accessed September 14, 2018, http://www.transplant
-observatory.org/organ-donation-transplantation-activities-2015-report-2/.

174 **the police burst in and arrested the couple:** Zofeen Ebrahim, "Organ Trafficking Resurfaces in Pakistan," IPS News Agency, August 27, 2012, http://
www.ipsnews.net/2012/08/organ-trafficking-resurfaces-in-pakistan/.

174 **A 2014 UNESCO report:** International Bioethics Committee, "Report of the
IBC on the Principle of Non-Discrimination and Non-Stigmatization," March
6, 2014, p. 18, http://unesdoc.unesco.org/images/0022/002211/221196E.pdf.

176 **Whether a regulated market in kidneys would be neutral:** Mahoney, "Altruism, Markets," 25.

176 **Small pilot studies:** Lee Bolton, "OPTN/UNOS: Public Comment Proposal—
A White Paper Addressing Financial Incentives for Organ Donation," accessed
September 14, 2018, https://optn.transplant.hrsa.gov/media/2084/Ethics_
PCProposal_Financial_Incentives_201701.pdf.

Seven: HUMAN EXPERIMENTS

183 **reckless with their patients:** Jonathan D. Moreno, Ulf Schmidt, and Steve
Joffe, "The Nuremberg Code 70 Years Later," *JAMA* 318, no. 9 (2017): 795–96.

184 **"this is no mere murder trial":** *Trials of War Criminals before the Nuernberg
Military Tribunals, Vol. 1* (Washington, DC: U.S. Government Printing Office,
1949), 27.

184 **White House–sponsored malaria experiment:** "Prison Malaria: Convicts
Expose Themselves to Disease so Doctors Can Study It," *Life Magazine*, June 4,
1945, 43–46.

185 **very strict and specific conditions:** Lawrence O. Gostin, Cori Vanchieri,
and Andrew Pope, eds., *Ethical Considerations for Research Involving Prisoners*
(Washington, DC: National Academies Press, 2007).

185 **The first line of the code:** The Nuremberg Code, accessed September 14, 2018,
https://history.nih.gov/research/downloads/nuremberg.pdf.

185 **U.S. newspapers as it unfolded:** Rothman, *Strangers*, 62.

186 **Jay Katz recalled the reactions:** Jay Katz, "The Consent Principle of the
Nuremberg Code: Its Significance Then and Now," in *The Nazi Doctors and
the Nuremberg Code: Human Rights in Human Experimentation*, eds. George J.
Annas and Michael A. Grodin (New York: Oxford University Press, 1992), 228.

186 **published in small print:** Jon M. Harkness, "Nuremberg and the Issue of Wartime Experiments on US Prisoners: The Green Committee," *JAMA* 276, no.
20 (1996): 1672–75; *see also* Dwight H. Green, "Ethics Governing the Service

of Prisoners as Subjects in Medical Experiments," *JAMA* 136, no. 7 (1948): 457–58.

187 **"there appears no question about the basic facts":** As quoted in Vincent J. Kopp, "Henry Knowles Beecher and the Development of Informed Consent in Anesthesia Research," *Anesthesiology* 90, no. 6 (1999): 1756–65.

187 **sure to erupt at some point:** Henry K. Beecher, "Experimentation in Man," *JAMA* 169 (1959): 461–78; *see also* Henry K. Beecher, "Ethics and Experimental Therapy," *JAMA* 186 (1963): 858–59.

187 **stunned the medical world:** Henry K. Beecher, "Ethics and Clinical Research," *New England Journal of Medicine* 274 (1966): 1354–60; for more information, *see* David S. Jones, Christine Grady, and Susan E. Lederer, " 'Ethics and Clinical Research'—The 50th Anniversary of Beecher's Bombshell," *New England Journal of Medicine* 374, no. 24 (June 2016): 2393–98.

188 **"were used as guinea pigs":** James P. McCaffrey, "Hospital Accused on Cancer Study; Live Cells Given to Patients without Their Consent, Director Tells Court; Allegation Is Denied; Chronic Disease Institution Defends Action—Value of Tests Is Praised," *New York Times*, January 21, 1964, 31, 51.

188 **Dr. Southam argued:** Allen M. Hornblum, "NYC's Forgotten Cancer Scandal," *New York Post*, December 28, 2013, https://nypost.com/2013/12/28/nycs -forgotten-cancer-scandal/.

188 **Saul Krugman began clinical studies:** Walter M. Robinson and Brandon T. Unruh, "The Hepatitis Experiments at the Willowbrook State School," in *The Oxford Textbook of Clinical Research Ethics*, eds. Ezekiel J. Emanuel et al. (New York: Oxford University Press, 2008), 80–85; *see also* Saul Krugman, "The Willowbrook Hepatitis Studies Revisited: Ethical Aspects," *Reviews of Infectious Diseases* 8, no. 1 (1986): 157–62.

190 **the *New York Times* reported:** Jean Heller, "Syphilis Victims in U.S. Study Went Untreated for 40 Years," *New York Times*, July 26, 1972, 1.

190 **a blue-ribbon panel:** *Final Report of the Tuskegee Syphilis Study Ad Hoc Advisory Panel*, April 28, 1973, http://www.research.usf.edu/dric/hrpp/foundations -course/docs/finalreport-tuskegeestudyadvisorypanel.pdf.

190 **enslaved persons for experimentation:** Todd Savitt, "The Use of Blacks for Medical Experimentation and Demonstration in the Old South," *Journal of Southern History* 48, no. 3 (1982): 331–48.

191 **mostly black Holmesburg Prison:** Allen M. Hornblum, *Acres of Skin: Human Experiments at Holmesburg Prison* (New York: Routledge, 1999).

191 **influential reports and recommendations:** For example, *see The Belmont Report*, https://www.hhs.gov/ohrp/regulations-and-policy/belmont-report/read -the-belmont-report/index.html.

191 **"resulting from a doctor's mixed emotions of compassion and ambitions":** Jerome Groopman, "The Elusive Artificial Heart," *New York Review of Books*, November 22, 2018, 25.

192 **Working exhaustively for eighteen months:** *Advisory Committee on Human Radiation Experiments—Final Report*, accessed September 14, 2018, https://ehss .energy.gov/ohre/roadmap/achre/report.html.

193 **Reverby was following up:** Reverby revealed her work first in a presentation: Susan M. Reverby, "'Normal Exposure' and Inoculation Syphilis: PHS 'Tuskegee,' Doctors in Guatemala, 1946–48 and at Sing Sing Prison, Ossining, New York, 1953–54" (May 2, 2010). Paper presented at the annual meeting of the American Association for the History of Medicine, Mayo Clinic, Rochester, MN. She published it later: "'Normal Exposure' and Inoculation Syphilis: A PHS 'Tuskegee' Doctor in Guatemala, 1946–48," *Journal of Policy History* 23 (2011): 6–28.

194 **One purpose:** Presidential Commission for the Study of Bioethical Issues, *Ethically Impossible: STD Research in Guatemala from 1946 to 1948* (Washington, DC, 2011), https://bioethicsarchive.georgetown.edu/pcsbi/sites/default/files/Ethically%20Impossible%20(with%20linked%20historical%20documents)%202.7.13.pdf.

196 **The FDA found that measurements of Jesse's liver:** "FDA's Notice of Initiation of Disqualification Proceeding and Opportunity to Explain," November 30, 2000, https://www.fda.gov/downloads/RegulatoryInformation/FOI/ElectronicReadingRoom/UCM144493.pdf.

196 **in the experimental treatment:** Robin Fretwell Wilson, "The Death of Jesse Gelsinger: New Evidence of the Influence of Money and Prestige in Human Research," *American Journal of Law and Medicine* 36 (2010): 295–325.

197 **The bipartisan 1980 Bayh-Dole Act:** Patent and Trademark Law Amendments Act (Bayh-Dole Act) of 1980, Pub. L. No. 96-517, 94 Stat. 3015 (codified as amended at 35 U.S.C. §§ 200-12 [2012]).

199 **the institutional complexities:** For meeting the institutional challenge of ensuring that individuals take responsibility when "many hands" are involved in pursuing a desired outcome, *see* Dennis F. Thompson, "The Problem of Many Hands," *American Political Science Review* 74, no. 4 (1980): 905–16.

199 **headline-grabbing results:** David L. Porter et al., "Chimeric Antigen Receptor-Modified T Cells in Chronic Lymphoid Leukemia," *New England Journal of Medicine* 365, no. 8 (August 2011): 725–33.

199 **A clinical trial at the Children's Hospital:** Shannon L. Maude et al., "Chimeric Antigen Receptor T Cells for Sustained Remissions in Leukemia," *New England Journal of Medicine* 371 (October 2014): 1507–17.

200 **As the FDA reasoned:** FDA News Release, "FDA Approval Brings First Gene Therapy to the United States," August 30, 2017, https://www.fda.gov/NewsEvents/Newsroom/PressAnnouncements/ucm574058.htm; "Dr. Scott Gottlieb Remarks on FDA Approval of First Gene Therapy in the United States," August 30, 2017, https://www.fda.gov/NewsEvents/Speeches/ucm574113.htm. A rigorous approval process should not be a needlessly duplicative one. In 2018 the NIH appropriately proposed streamlining the human gene therapy trials review system and putting greater emphasis on lab safety. Francis M. Collins and Scott Gottlieb, "The Next Phase of Human Gene-Therapy Oversight," *New England Journal of Medicine* 379, no. 15 (October 2018): 1393–95.

201 **As June put it:** Allysia Finley, "How HIV Became a Cancer Cure," *Wall Street Journal*, August 18, 2017, https://www.wsj.com/articles/how-hiv-became-a-cancer

-cure-1503092082. We share concerns about the prices charged by drug companies that are being developed by Carl June and others. At least one analysis indicates that the high prices are not justified by the actual production costs. Ezekiel J. Emanuel, "We Can't Afford the Drugs That Could Cure Cancer," *Wall Street Journal*, September 20, 2018, https://www.wsj.com/articles/we-cant-afford-the-drugs-that-could-cure-cancer-1537457740.

202 **"something" being an anthrax attack:** Presidential Commission for the Study of Bioethical Issues, Transcript, Meeting 9, Distinguished Speaker, May 17, 2012, https://bioethicsarchive.georgetown.edu/pcsbi/node/716.html.

203 **Two opposing sides lined up:** Some of the narrative comes from Amy Gutmann and James W. Wagner, "Reflections on Democratic Deliberation in Bioethics," special issue, *Hastings Center Report*, May/June 2017.

203 **the bioethics commission recommended an ethical way:** Presidential Commission for the Study of Bioethical Issues, *Safeguarding Children: Pediatric Medical Countermeasure Research* (Washington, DC, 2013).

Eight: REPRODUCTIVE TECHNOLOGIES

207 **custody case over "Baby M":** *In the Matter of Baby M, a Pseudonym for an Actual Person*, 109 N.J. 396, 537 A.2d 1227 (1988).

207 **a New Jersey court in 2009:** Ted Sherman, "N.J. Gay Couple Fight for Custody of Twin 5-Year-Old Girls," nj.com, December 20, 2011, https://www.nj.com/news/index.ssf/2011/12/nj_gay_couple_fight_for_custod.html.

209 **legal appeals in both India and Germany:** Yasmine Ergas, "Babies without Borders: Human Rights, Human Dignity, and the Regulation of International Commercial Surrogacy," *Emory International Law Review* 27 (2013): 117–88.

209 **children conceived by gestational surrogacy may be born legally stateless:** Ergas, "Babies without Borders," 188.

211 **embryos did not have rights to the estate:** Keith Dalton, "Dead Couple's Embryos to Be Thawed," *Washington Post*, December 4, 1987, https://www.washingtonpost.com/archive/politics/1987/12/04/dead-couples-embryos-to-be-thawed/53c4cacb-ab70-4f2b-86b1-c0ff72879da9/.

211 **the Tennessee Supreme Court found:** *Davis v. Davis*, 842 S.W.2d 588 (Tenn. 1992).

211 **an Arizona state law specified:** "Arizona Passes Law to Dictate How Separated Couples' Frozen Embryos Can Be Used," wbur.org, April 17, 2018, http://www.wbur.org/hereandnow/2018/04/17/arizona-frozen-embryos-law.

212 **embryos could become objects of manipulation:** For a general discussion of these issues, *see* Paul Lombardo, ed., *A Century of Eugenics in America: From the Indiana Experiment to the Human Genome Era* (Bloomington: Indiana University Press, 2011).

214 **first director general of UNESCO:** Julian Huxley, *Unesco: Its Purpose and Its Philosophy* (London: Frederick Printing, 1946), 38, http://unesdoc.unesco.org/images/0006/000681/068197eo.pdf.

214   **Hence the title of his 1974 book:** Joseph Fletcher, *The Ethics of Genetic Control: Ending Reproductive Roulette* (New York: Anchor Press/Doubleday, 1974).

215   **Princeton University theologian Paul Ramsey:** Paul Ramsey, *Fabricated Man: The Ethics of Genetic Control* (New Haven, CT: Yale University Press, 1970).

216   **"It hangs like a cloud":** Carl Zimmer, *She Has Her Mother's Laugh: The Powers, Perversions, and Potential of Heredity* (New York: Dutton, 2018).

216   **defenders of deaf culture:** Susannah Baruch, "Preimplantation Genetic Diagnosis and Parental Preferences: Beyond Deadly Disease," *Houston Journal of Health Law and Policy* 8 (2008): 245–70.

219   **Leon Kass has mourned the extinction:** Leon R. Kass, "The End of Courtship," American Enterprise Institute, September 23, 2002, https://www.aei.org/publication/the-end-of-courtship/.

219   **legal theorist Robert George:** Robert P. George, *In Defense of Natural Law* (Oxford: Oxford University Press, 2001).

220   **connection among marriage, sex, and procreation:** Sherif Girgis, Ryan T. Anderson, and Robert P. George, *What Is Marriage? Man and Woman: A Defense* (New York: Encounter Books, 2012), 36.

220   **Marriage that is "sealed or consummated":** Sherif Girgis, Ryan T. Anderson, and Robert P. George, "What Is Marriage?" *Harvard Journal of Law and Public Policy* 34, no. 1 (2010): 245–88.

220   **"loving union of mind and body":** Girgis et al., *What Is Marriage?*, 30.

220   **Stephen Macedo pinpoints its crux:** For the most comprehensive, respectful, and trenchant critique of the New Natural Law position on marriage, *see* Stephen Macedo, *Just Married: Same-Sex Couples, Monogamy & the Future of Marriage* (Princeton, NJ: Princeton University Press, 2015), 43.

224   **if the likely benefits are on balance worthwhile:** Sara Reardon, " 'Three-Parent Baby' Claim Raises Hope—and Ethical Concerns," *Nature*, September 29, 2016, https://www.nature.com/news/three-parent-baby-claim-raises-hopes-and-ethical-concerns-1.20698.

225   **committees in both the United States and the United Kingdom:** National Academies of Science, Engineering, and Medicine, *Mitochondrial Replacement Techniques: Ethical, Social, and Policy Considerations* (Washington, DC: National Academies Press, 2016), 123; *see also* Human Fertilisation and Embryology Authority, "UK's Independent Expert Panel Recommends 'Cautious Adoption' of Mitochondrial Donation in Treatment," October 10, 2017, https://www.hfea.gov.uk/about-us/news-and-press-releases/2016-news-and-press-releases/uks-independent-expert-panel-recommends-cautious-adoption-of-mitochondrial-donation-in-treatment/.

Nine: OPENING CELL DOORS

227   **Rebecca Skloot's riveting history:** Rebecca Skloot, *The Immortal Life of Henrietta Lacks* (New York: Broadway Books, 2011).

228 **Moore sued on the grounds:** *Moore v. Regents of University of California*, 51 Cal. 3d 120, 793 P.2d 479 (1990).

229 **That feat was accomplished by two labs in 1998:** James A. Thomson et al., "Embryonic Stem Cell Lines Derived from Human Blastocysts," *Science* 282, no. 5391 (November 1998): 1145–47; Michael J. Shamblott et al., "Derivation of Pluripotent Stem Cells from Cultured Human Primordial Germ Cells," *PNAS* 95, no. 23 (November 1998): 13726–31.

230 **a sheep they called Dolly:** Accessed September 14, 2018, http://dolly.roslin.ed .ac.uk/facts/the-life-of-dolly/index.html.

230 **The first successful cloning of primates:** Ben Guarino, "Researchers Clone the First Primates from Monkey Tissue Cells," *Washington Post*, January 24, 2018, https://www.washingtonpost.com/news/speaking-of-science/wp/2018/01/24/ researchers-clone-the-first-primates-from-monkey-tissue-cells/?utm_term= .fbe9f502d253.

231 **President Clinton announced a ban:** Rick Weiss, "Clinton Forbids Funding of Human Clone Studies," *Washington Post*, March 5, 1997, https://www .washingtonpost.com/archive/politics/1997/03/05/clinton-forbids-funding-of -human-clone-studies/3b2f831f-f23e-4457-8611-6c9bda0b8ebf/.

231 **Bush declared that he would permit no more federal funding:** George W. Bush White House Archives, "President Discusses Stem Cell Research," August 9, 2001, https://georgewbush-whitehouse.archives.gov/news/releases/ 2001/08/20010809-2.html.

232 **Leon Kass, was a trenchant critic:** Leon R. Kass, "Reflections on Public Bioethics: A View from the Trenches," *Kennedy Institute of Ethics Journal* 15, no. 3 (2005): 221–50.

232 **States like California and New York:** Ruchir N. Karmali, Natalie M. Jones, and Aaron D. Levine, "Tracking and Assessing the Rise of State-Funded Stem Cell Research," *Nature Biotechnology* 28, no. 12 (2010): 1246–48; *see also* National Research Council and Institute of Medicine of the National Academies, *Guidelines for Human Embryonic Stem Cell Research* (Washington, DC: National Academies Press, 2005), 75.

233 **Surveys show that since the late 1970s:** Evan Lehmann, "Conservatives Lose Faith in Science over Last 40 Years," *Scientific American*, March 30, 2012, https://www.scientificamerican.com/article/conservatives-lose-faith-in-science -over-last-40-years/.

233 **we are all living in embryoville:** Kass, "Reflections on Public Bioethics," 223.

233 **an academy committee made a series of recommendations:** National Research Council, *Guidelines*, 99–102, 105–6.

234 **In his 2006 State of the Union address:** George W. Bush White House, State of the Union address, January 31, 2006, https://georgewbush-whitehouse .archives.gov/stateoftheunion/2006/.

234 **the bill would have prohibited the creation of a whole range of human-nonhuman organisms:** S.1435 Human-Animal Hybrid Prohibition Act of 2009, 111th Congress (2009–2010), accessed September 14, 2018, https://www .congress.gov/bill/111th-congress/senate-bill/1435/text.

235 **The underlying worry was that creating lab animals with a mixture of human and nonhuman parts:** Jonathan D. Moreno, "Why We Need to Be More Accepting of 'Humanized' Lab Animals," *Atlantic*, October 2011, https://www.theatlantic.com/health/archive/2011/10/why-we-need-to-be-more -accepting-of-humanized-lab-animals/246071/.

235 **backed up by survey evidence:** Alison Abbott, "Regulations Proposed for Animal-Human Chimaeras," *Nature* 475 (2011): 438.

236 **In 2007 a Japanese lab reported:** Kazutoshi Takahashi et al., "Induction of Pluripotent Stem Cells from Adult Human Fibroblasts by Defined Factors," *Cell* 131, no. 5 (November 2007): 861–72. Around the same time, another team, led by Thomson, made the same discovery: Junying Yu et al., "Induced Pluripotent Stem Cell Lines Derived from Human Somatic Cells," *Science* 318, no. 5858 (December 2007): 1917–20.

236 **McCain had also pointed out:** Rich Klein and Jennifer Parker, "Politics of Stem Cell Debate in Flux," abcnews.go.com, June 20, 2007, https://abcnews.go .com/Politics/story?id=3297955&page=1.

237 **When Barack Obama took office:** Obama Executive Order 13505, accessed September 14, 2018, https://www.gpo.gov/fdsys/pkg/DCPD-200900136/ content-detail.html; https://www.gpo.gov/fdsys/pkg/FR-2009-03-11/pdf/E9 -5441.pdf; *see also* Sheryl Gay Stolberg, "Obama Is Leaving Some Stem Cell Issues to Congress," *New York Times*, March 8, 2009, https://www.nytimes .com/2009/03/09/us/politics/09stem.html.

237 **the mechanism of the Zika virus:** Jonathan D. Moreno, "How a Zika Virus Breakthrough Vindicates Stem Cell Research," *HuffPost*, March 16, 2017, https://www.huffingtonpost.com/jonathan-d-moreno/how-a-zika-virus -breakthr_b_9472846.html.

238 **the J. Craig Venter Institute in Maryland:** Daniel G. Gibson et al., "Creation of a Bacterial Cell Controlled by a Chemically Synthesized Genome," *Science* 329, no. 5987 (July 2010): 52–56.

238 **President Obama asked his Presidential Commission:** Note that we take some language here directly from the report coauthored with the commission, but the opinions expressed here are our own and we are not more generally representing the commission. Presidential Commission for the Study of Bioethical Issues, *New Directions: The Ethics of Synthetic Biology and Emerging Technologies* (Washington, DC: 2010), accessed September 14, 2018, https://bioethicsarchive .georgetown.edu/pcsbi/sites/default/files/PCSBI-Synthetic-Biology-Report-12 .16.10_0.pdf; letter from Obama to Gutmann reproduced at p. vi; quote is from "New Directions," p. 23, emphasis added.

239 **Those public deliberations gave voice to the widest range of viewpoints:** Presidential Commission for the Study of Bioethical Issues, "New Directions," 21.

239 **As two medical ethicists put their critique:** Joachim Boldt and Oliver Muller, "Newtons of the Leaves of Grass," *Nature Biotechnology* 26, no. 11 (2008): 387–89.

240 **one critic of biotechnology:** ETC Group, "Synthia Is Alive . . . and Breed-

ing: Panacea or Pandora's Box?," etcgroup.org, May 20, 2010, http://www
.etcgroup.org/content/synthia-alive-%E2%80%A6-and-breeding-panacea-or
-pandoras-box.

240 **One official of the Italian bishops' conference:** Jonathan D. Moreno, "The
First Scientist to 'Play God' Was Not Craig Venter," *Science Progress*, May 25,
2010, https://scienceprogress.org/2010/05/synbio-ethics/.

240 **Bonnie Bassler, who testified before:** Bonnie Bassler, testimony, Overview and
Context of the Science and Technology of Synthetic Biology (Washington, DC:
July 8, 2010), https://bioethicsarchive.georgetown.edu/pcsbi/node/164.html.

241 **"environment are astoundingly complex":** Presidential Commission for the
Study of Bioethical Issues, "New Directions," 22.

242 **In historic firsts for immunotherapy:** Kymriah approved August 30, 2017,
https://www.fda.gov/newsevents/newsroom/pressannouncements/ucm574058
.htm; Yescarta approved October 18, 2017, https://www.fda.gov/newsevents/
newsroom/pressannouncements/ucm581216.htm.

Immunotherapy remains a serious intervention whose risks are not fully
understood. Despite the impressive success in cases like that of Emily Whitehead, one patient with leukemia died after the experimental treatment because,
though his cancer-fighting cells were altered as planned, so was a leukemia cell.
That one cell multiplied and eventually caused his death. This rare and unanticipated event taught scientists about the destructive power of a single cell, but
at the highest cost imaginable. Denise Grady, "Breakthrough Leukemia Treatment Backfires in Rare Case," *New York Times*, October 1, 2018.

243 **Google has claimed that:** Miguel Helft, "Google Uses Searches to Track
Flu's Spread," *New York Times*, November 12, 2008, https://www.nytimes
.com/2008/11/12/technology/internet/12flu.html.

244 **At least one company has been formed:** Flatiron, accessed September 14,
2018, https://flatiron.com/about-us/.

244 **Britain's Nuffield Council on Bioethics has been among:** Nuffield Council
on Bioethics, *The Collection, Linking and Use of Data in Biomedical Research and
Health Care: Ethical Issues* (February 2015), 46–57.

245 **One careful study found that 40 percent of the results:** Stephany Tandy-
Connor et al., "False-Positive Results Released by Direct-to-Consumer Genetics
Tests Highlight the Importance of Clinical Confirmation Testing for Appropri-
ate Patient Care," *Genetics in Medicine* (2018), doi:10.1038/gim.2018.38

245 **An FDA officer noted, however:** U.S. Food & Drug Administration, "FDA
Allows Marketing of First Direct-to-Consumer Tests That Provide Genetic
Risk Information for Certain Conditions, April 6, 2017. https://www.fda.gov/
NewsEvents/Newsroom/PressAnnouncements/ucm551185.htm.

245 **23andMe is reported to have the largest biobank:** Antonio Regalado,
"23andMe Sells Data for Drug Search," *MIT Technology Review*, June 21, 2016,
https://www.technologyreview.com/s/601506/23andme-sells-data-for-drug
-search/.

246 **"separate express consent":** "Privacy Best Practices for Consumer Genetic
Testing Services," Future of Privacy Forum, July 31, 2018, https://fpf.org/

wp-content/uploads/2018/07/Privacy-Best-Practices-for-Consumer-Genetic
-Testing-Services-FINAL.pdf.

246 **just a bit of digging into publicly available:** Erika Check Hayden, "Privacy Protections: The Genome Hacker," *Nature* 497 (2016): 172–74.

246 **The captivating story featured the detective and DNA expert:** Justin Jouvenal, "To Find Alleged Golden State Killer, Investigators First Found His Great-Great-Great Grandparents," *Washington Post*, April 30, 2018, https://www .washingtonpost.com/local/public-safety/to-find-alleged-golden-state-killer -investigators-first-found-his-great-great-great-grandparents/2018/04/30/3c86 5fe7-dfcc-4a0e-b6b2-0bec548d501f_story.html.

247 **when the Human Genome Project got started:** Accessed September 14, 2018, https://www.genome.gov/10001618/the-elsi-research-program/.

247 **has come to be called gene editing:** Eric S. Lander, "The Heroes of CRISPR," *Cell* 164 (2016): 24–25.

248 **rigorous regulatory standards:** National Academies of Sciences, Engineering, and Medicine, "Human Genome Editing" (Washington, DC: National Academies Press, 2017).

250 **involves editing the germ line:** Dietram A. Scheufele et al., "U.S. Attitudes on Human Genome Editing," *Science* 357, no. 6351 (August 2017): 553–54.

250 **a team in China reported:** Kat Eschner, "Scientists 'Went Rogue' and Genetically Engineered Two Human Babies—or at Least Claimed to," *Popular Science*, November 26, 2018, https://www.popsci.com/crispr-twin-babies -genetic-engineering.

250 **thought of themselves as an "invisible college":** Caroline S. Wagner, *The New Invisible College* (Washington, D.C.: Brookings Institution Press, 2008).

250 **many ethical issues will need to be addressed:** For example, *see* Amy Gutmann and Jonathan D. Moreno, "Keep CRISPR Safe: Regulating a Genetic Revolution," *Foreign Affairs* (May/June 2018), 171–76.

Epilogue: TRANSFORMING MINDS

253 **Oliver Sacks's book about L-dopa:** Oliver Sacks, *Awakenings*, reprint ed. (New York: Vintage, 1999).

254 **give feedback to our brains:** Emily B. Falk and Danielle S. Bassett, "Brain and Social Networks: Fundamental Building Blocks of Human Experience," *Trends in Cognitive Science* 21, no. 9 (2017): 674–90.

254 **including high-risk adolescents:** Scholars have explored how findings in developmental neuroscience could inform legal regimes that implicate the unique decision-making vulnerabilities of adolescents. *See* Michael N. Tennison and Amanda C. Pustilnik, "'And If Your Friends Jumped Off a Bridge, Would You Do It Too?' How Developmental Neuroscience Can Inform Legal Regimes Governing Adolescents," *Indiana Health Law Review* 12, no. 2 (2015): 534–85.

254 **In the case of seat belts:** Philip H. Dougherty, "Advertising; Seat Belt Campaign and Law," *New York Times*, November 30, 1984, D19; *see also* Joseph

Berger, "Deaths Drop 27% with State's Seat-Belt Law," *New York Times*, May 1, 1985, A1.

255 **we cannot maximize all that we value:** Ruth Faden, "Ethical Issues in Government Sponsored Public Health Campaigns," *Health Education Quarterly* 14, no. 1 (1987): 27–37.

255 **with the way their brains respond:** Three messages from an e-mail campaign sponsored by the New York State Smokers' Quitline were "Stop Smoking. Start Living," coupled with negative or neutral images; or "What Are the Good Things That Would Happen If You Quit Smoking?" coupled with neutral images; or "What Are the Bad Things That Would Happen If You Don't Stop Smoking?" coupled with negative images. *See* Emily B. Falk et al., "Functional Brain Imaging Predicts Public Health Campaign Success," *Social Cognitive and Affective Neuroscience* 11, no. 2 (February 2016): 204–14; *see also* Emily B. Falk et al., "Predicting Persuasion-Induced Behavior Change from the Brain," *Journal of Neuroscience* 30, no. 25 (June 2010): 8421–24.

257 **Vance Packard wrote a best seller:** Vance Packard, *The Hidden Persuaders*, reissue ed. (New York: IG, 2007).

258 **EEG measurements while people are shopping:** Natasha Singer, "Making Ads That Whisper to the Brain," *New York Times*, November 13, 2010, https://www.nytimes.com/2010/11/14/business/14stream.html.

258 **deliberately manipulated the news feeds:** Vindu Goel, "Facebook Tinkers with Users' Emotions in News Feed Experiment, Stirring Outcry," *New York Times*, June 30, 2014, https://www.nytimes.com/2014/06/30/technology/facebook-tinkers-with-users-emotions-in-news-feed-experiment-stirring-outcry.html.

259 **responding to a certain brand:** Rotterdam School of Management, Erasmus University, RSM Discovery (blog), *Identifying Strong Brands in the Brain*, June 8, 2018, https://discovery.rsm.nl/articles/detail/348-strong-brands-can-be-identified-in-the-brain/.

260 **Generally speaking, the standard of responsibility:** Nita Farahany and James E. Coleman Jr. "Genetics, Neuroscience, and Criminal Responsibility," in *The Impact of the Behavioral Sciences on Criminal Law*, ed. Nita Farahany (Oxford: Oxford University Press, 2009). Farahany and Coleman make the important point that demonstrating brain injury disposition to crime is a double-edged sword: it can be used to argue for the social value of imprisonment for people disposed to violent criminality.

261 **they don't depend on brain scans:** In some cases of individuals convicted of heinous crimes, psychologist Adrian Raine has used a combination of biographical details of an abusive childhood, psychometric tests, and brain scans showing gross anatomical defects to urge courts to reduce a penalty from death to life in prison without parole. We would note, however, that the same evidence of brain defects predisposing someone to heinous crime also can be used to argue, from a deterrence perspective, against punishment shorter than life imprisonment. *See* Adrian Raine, *The Anatomy of Violence: The Biological Roots of Crime* (New York: Random House 2013).

262 **law professor Hank Greely:** Henry T. Greely et al., "Thinking about the Human Neuron Mouse," *American Journal of Bioethics* 7, no. 5 (May 2007): 27–40.

262 **But the ethical issues about experiments with brain tissue:** Nita A. Farahany, et al., "The Ethics of Experimenting with Human Brain Tissue," *Nature* 556 (April 26, 2018): 429–32.

263 **"a pretty girl or a carefully wired robot":** Alvin Toffler, *Future Shock* (New York: Bantam, 1984), 211.

264 **in his book *Musicophilia*:** Oliver Sacks, *Musicophilia: Tales of Music and the Brain* (New York: Knopf, 2007).

264 **neuroscientist Eric Kandel recalls:** Eric R. Kandel, *In Search of Memory: The Emergence of a New Science of Mind* (New York: W. W. Norton, 2006).

265 **people with diseases like epilepsy:** Youssef Ezzyat et al., "Closed-Loop Stimulation of Temporal Cortex Rescues Functional Networks and Improves Memory," *Nature Communications* 9, no. 1 (February 2018): 365.

265 **studies have yielded disappointing results:** Joachim C. Burbiel, "Primary Prevention of Posttraumatic Stress Disorder: Drugs and Implications," *Military Medical Research* 2 (2015): 24.

267 **one in twenty-four women will be diagnosed with it:** Steven Nurkin, "Symptoms of Colon Cancer in Women," RoswellPark.org, March 23, 2018, https://www.roswellpark.org/cancertalk/201803/symptoms-colon-cancer-women.

267 **Eva recounts in her moving memoir, *Good Beyond Evil*:** Eva Gossman, *Good Beyond Evil: Ordinary People in Extraordinary Times* (London: Vallentine Mitchell, 2002).

268 **Herceptin is extremely expensive but found to be cost-effective:** Louis P. Garrison, Jr., et al., "Cost-Effectiveness Analysis of Trastuzumab in the Adjuvant Setting for Treatment of HER2-Positive Breast Cancer," Cancer 110, no. 3 (August 1, 2007): 489-498.

BIBLIOGRAPHY

Abbott, Alison. "Regulations Proposed for Animal-Human Chimaeras." *Nature* 475 (2011): 438.

"Achievements in Public Health, 1900–1999: Fluoridation of Drinking Water to Prevent Dental Caries." *MMWR* 48, no. 41 (October 1999): 933–40.

Adams, Tim. "How to Spot a Murderer's Brain." *Guardian*, May 12, 2013. https://www.theguardian.com/science/2013/may/12/how-to-spot-a-murderers-brain.

Advisory Committee on Human Radiation Experiments—Final Report. Accessed September 14, 2018. https://ehss.energy.gov/ohre/roadmap/achre/report.html.

Alexander, Shana. "They Decide Who Lives, Who Dies." *Life Magazine*, November 9, 1962.

Anderson, Gerard, Uwe E. Reinhardt, Peter S. Hussey, and Varduhi Petrosyan. "It's the Prices, Stupid: Why the United States Is So Different from Other Countries." *Health Affairs* 22, no. 3 (May–June 2003): 89–105.

Antommaria, Armand Matheny. "'Who Should Survive? One of the Choices on Our Conscience': Mental Retardation and the History of Contemporary Bioethics." *Kennedy Institute of Ethics Journal* 16, no. 3 (September 2006): 205–24.

"Arizona Passes Law to Dictate How Separated Couples' Frozen Embryos Can Be Used." wbur.org, April 17, 2018. http://www.wbur.org/hereandnow/2018/04/17/arizona-frozen-embryos-law.

Arrow, Kenneth J. "Uncertainty and the Welfare Economics of Medical Care." *American Economic Review* 53, no. 5 (1963): 941–73.

Aviv, Rachel. "What Does It Mean to Die?," *New Yorker*, February 5, 2018. https://www.newyorker.com/magazine/2018/02/05/what-does-it-mean-to-die.

Bächtiger, André, John S. Dryzek, Jane Mansbridge, and Mark E. Warren. *The Oxford Handbook of Deliberative Democracy.* Oxford: Oxford University Press, 2018.

Baruch, Susannah. "Preimplantation Genetic Diagnosis and Parental Preferences: Beyond Deadly Disease." *Houston Journal of Health Law and Policy* 8 (2008): 245–70.

Bassler, Bonnie. Testimony before the Presidential Commission for the Study of Bioethical Issues: "Overview and Context of the Science and Technology of Synthetic Biology." Washington, DC, July 8, 2010. https://bioethicsarchive.georgetown.edu/pcsbi/node/164.html.

Beauchamp, Tom L., and James F. Childress. *Principles of Biomedical Ethics.* New York: Oxford University Press, 2012.

Beecher, Henry K. "Ethics and Clinical Research." *New England Journal of Medicine* 274 (1966): 1354–60.

———. "Ethics and Experimental Therapy." *JAMA* 186 (1963): 858–59.

———. "Experimentation in Man." *JAMA* 169 (1959): 461–78.

———. "The Powerful Placebo." *JAMA* 159, no. 17 (1955): 1602–6.

Bentham, Jeremy. *Rights, Representation, and Reform: Nonsense upon Stilts and Other Writings on the French Revolution.* Edited by Philip Schofield, Catherine Pease-Watkin, and Cyprian Blamires. New York: Oxford University Press, 2002.

Berg, Paul. "Asilomar 1975: DNA Modification Secured." *Nature* 455 (2008): 290–91.

Berger, Joseph. "Deaths Drop 27% with State's Seat-Belt Law." *New York Times*, May 1, 1985, A1.

Bernstein, Lenny. "U.S. Life Expectancy Declines Again, A Dismal Trend Not Seen Since World War I." *Washington Post*, November 29, 2018. https://www .washingtonpost.com/national/health-science/us-life-expectancy-declines-again -a-dismal-trend-not-seen-since-world-war-i/2018/11/28/ae58bc8c-f28c-11e8-bc79 -68604ed88993_story.html?utm_term=.7fcf78ee8356.

———. "U.S. Life Expectancy Declines for the First Time since 1993." *Washington Post*, December 8, 2016. https://www.washingtonpost.com/national/ health-science/us-life-expectancy-declines-for-the-first-time-since-1993/2016/ 12/07/7dcdc7b4-bc93-11e6-91ee-1adddfe36cbe_story.html?utm_term=.181fa 1dc4e55.

Bersoff, Donald N. 2013 Presidential Address to the American Psychological Association. Described in Donald N. Bersoff, "Protecting Victims of Violent Patients While Protecting Confidentiality." *American Psychologist* 69, no. 5 (2013): 461–67.

Blendon, Robert, John M. Benson, and Joachim O. Hero. "Public Trust in Physicians: U.S. Medicine in International Perspective." *New England Journal of Medicine* 371, no. 17 (October 2014): 1570–72.

Boldt, Joachim, and Oliver Muller. "Newtons of the Leaves of Grass." *Nature Biotechnology* 26, no. 11 (2008): 387–89.

Bollyky, Thomas J., Aaron S. Kesselheim, and Joshua M. Sharfstein. "What Trump Should Actually Do about the High Cost of Drugs." *New York Times*, May 14, 2018. https://www.nytimes.com/2018/05/14/opinion/trump-costs-drugs-pricing .html.

Bolton, Lee. "OPTN/UNOS: Public Comment Proposal—A White Paper Addressing Financial Incentives for Organ Donation." Accessed September 14, 2018. https://optn.transplant.hrsa.gov/media/2084/Ethics_PCProposal_Financial_ Incentives_201701.pdf.

Brody, Jane. "25 Years of Fluoride Cuts Tooth Decay in Newburgh." *New York Times*, May 3, 1970, L64.

Bromwich, David. *The Intellectual Life of Edmund Burke: From the Sublime and the Beautiful to American Independence.* Cambridge, MA: Belknap Press, 2014.

Brooks, David, and Gail Collins. "The Conversation: What Would Edmund Burke Say?" *New York Times*, October 21, 2014. https://opinionator.blogs.nytimes .com/2014/10/21/what-would-edmund-burke-say/.

Burbiel, Joachim C. "Primary Prevention of Posttraumatic Stress Disorder: Drugs and Implications." *Military Medical Research* 2 (2015): 24.

Bush, George W. "President Discusses Stem Cell Research." August 9, 2001. https:// georgewbush-whitehouse.archives.gov/news/releases/2001/08/20010809-2.html.

———. "State of the Union 2006." https://georgewbush-whitehouse.archives.gov/ stateoftheunion/2006/.

Callahan, Sidney, and Daniel Callahan, eds. *Abortion: Understanding Differences.* New York: Springer, 1984.

Caplan, Arthur. "Bioethics of Organ Transplantation." *Cold Spring Harbor Perspectives in Medicine* 4, no. 3 (March 2014), a015685.

Capron, Alexander M., and Francis L. Delmonico. "Cover the Costs for Kidney Donors to Increase the Supply." *New York Times*, August 22, 2014. https://www .nytimes.com/roomfordebate/2014/08/21/how-much-for-a-kidney/cover-the -costs-for-kidney-donors-to-increase-the-supply.

Carroll, Aaron E., and Austin Frakt. "Save Lives. It Can Save Money. So Why Aren't We Spending More on Public Health?" *New York Times*, May 28, 2018. https:// www.nytimes.com/2018/05/28/upshot/it-saves-lives-it-can-save-money-so-why -arent-we-spending-more-on-public-health.html.

Case, Anne, and Angus Deaton. "Rising Morbidity and Mortality in Midlife among White Non-Hispanic Americans in the 21st Century." *PNAS* 112, no. 49 (December 2015): 15078–83.

Cavallo, Jo. "Debate over Legalizing Physician-Assisted Death for the Terminally Ill." *ASCO Post*, December 15, 2014. http://www.ascopost.com/issues/december-15 -2014/debate-over-legalizing-physician-assisted-death-for-the-terminally-ill/.

Centers for Disease Control and Prevention. "National Antimicrobial Resistance Monitoring System for Enteric Bacteria (NARMS)." Accessed September 14, 2018. https://www.cdc.gov/narms/faq.html.

Childress, James F., and Cathryn T. Liverman, eds. "Organ Donation—Opportunities for Action: Committee on Increasing Rates of Organ Donation, Board on Health Sciences Policy." Washington, DC: National Academies Press, 2006.

Chokshi, Neel P., Srinath Adusumalli, Dylan S. Small, Alexander Morris, Jordyn Feingold, YoonHee P. Ha, Charles A. Rareshide, Victoria Hilbert, and Mitesh S. Patel. "Loss-Framed Financial Incentives and Personalized Goal-Setting to Increase Physical Activity among Ischemic Heart Disease Patients Using Wearable Devices: The ACTIVE REWARD Randomized Trial." *Journal of the American Heart Association* 7, no. 12 (June 2018): e009173.

Collins, Francis M., and Scott Gottlieb. "The Next Phase of Human Gene-Therapy Oversight." *New England Journal of Medicine* 379, no. 15 (October 11, 2018): 1393–95.

Commonwealth Fund. "New 11-Country Study: U.S. Health Care System Has Widest Gap between People with Higher and Lower Incomes." July 2017.

Courtemanche, Charles J., and Daniel Zapata, "Does Universal Coverage Improve Health? The Massachusetts Experience." NBER Working Paper Number 17893, Cambridge, MA: National Bureau of Economic Research, 2014. https://www .nber.org/papers/w17893.

Cutler, David, and Steven M. Walsh. "The Massachusetts Target on Medical Spending

Growth." *NEJM Catalyst*, May 11, 2016. https://catalyst.nejm.org/massachusetts
-target-medical-spending-growth/.

Dalton, Keith. "Dead Couple's Embryos to Be Thawed." *Washington Post*, December 4, 1987. https://www.washingtonpost.com/archive/politics/1987/12/04/dead
-couples-embryos-to-be-thawed/53c4cacb-ab70-4f2b-86b1-c0ff72879da9/.

Daniels, Norman. "Equity of Access to Health Care: Some Conceptual and Ethical
Issues." Paper delivered to the President's Commission for the Study of Ethical
Issues in Medicine and Biomedical and Behavioral Research, Washington, DC,
March 13, 1981.

———. *Just Health Care*. Cambridge: Cambridge University Press, 1985.

Dax's Case, produced by Unicorn Media, Inc. for Concern for Dying (1985), DVD.

de Beauvoir, Simone. *A Very Easy Death*. Translated by Patrick O'Brian. New York:
Pantheon Books, 1965. Originally published as *Une mort très douce*. Paris: Gallimard, 1964.

Deer, Brian. "Andrew Wakefield: The Fraud Investigation." Accessed September 14,
2008. https://briandeer.com/mmr/lancet-summary.htm.

"A Definition of Irreversible Coma: Report of the Ad Hoc Committee of the Harvard
Medical School to Examine the Definition of Brain Death." *JAMA* 205, no. 6
(1968): 337–40.

Deggans, Eric. " 'Nurse Jackie' Ends as TV's Most Honest Depiction of Addiction."
NPR, April 12, 2015. https://www.npr.org/2015/04/10/398713112/nurse-jackie
-ends-as-tvs-most-honest-depiction-of-addiction.

Dickman, Samuel L., Steffie Woolhandler, Jacob Bor, Danny McCormick, David H.
Bor, and David U. Himmelstein. "Health Spending for Low-, Middle-, and High-
Income Americans, 1963–2012." *Health Affairs* 35, no. 7 (July 2016): 1189–96.

Dougherty, Philip H. "Advertising; Seat Belt Campaign and Law." *New York Times*,
November 30, 1984, D19.

Downs, David. "The Science behind the DEA's Long War on Marijuana." *Scientific
American*, April 19, 2016. https://www.scientificamerican.com/article/the-science
-behind-the-dea-s-long-war-on-marijuana/.

Ebrahim, Zofeen. "Organ Trafficking Resurfaces in Pakistan." IPS News Agency,
August 27, 2012. http://www.ipsnews.net/2012/08/organ-trafficking-resurfaces
-in-pakistan/.

Editorial. "Want Reliable Medical Information? The Trump Administration Doesn't."
New York Times, July 19, 2018. https://www.nytimes.com/2018/07/19/opinion/
trump-medicine-data-hhs-ahrq.html.

Emanuel, Ezekiel J. "The Real Cost of the US Health Care System." *JAMA* 319, no.
10 (2018): 983–85.

———. "We Can't Afford the Drugs That Could Cure Cancer." *Wall Street Journal*,
September 20, 2018. https://www.wsj.com/articles/we-cant-afford-the-drugs-that
-could-cure-cancer-1537457740.

Emanuel, Ezekiel J., Bregje D. Onwuteaka-Philipsen, John W. Urwin, and Joachim
Cohen. "Attitudes and Practices of Euthanasia and Physician-Assisted Suicide in
the United States, Canada, and Europe." *JAMA* 316, no. 1 (July 2016): 79–90.

Ergas, Yasmine. "Babies without Borders: Human Rights, Human Dignity, and the

Regulation of International Commercial Surrogacy." *Emory International Law Review* 27 (2013): 117–88.

Eschner, Kat. "Scientists 'Went Rogue' and Genetically Engineered Two Human Babies—or at Least Claimed to." *Popular Science*, November 26, 2018. https://www.popsci.com/crispr-twin-babies-genetic-engineering.

ETC Group. "Synthia Is Alive . . . and Breeding: Panacea or Pandora's Box?," etc group.org, May 20, 2010. http://www.etcgroup.org/content/synthia-alive-%E2%80%A6-and-breeding-panacea-or-pandoras-box.

"Expanding Access to Investigational Therapies for HIV Infection and AIDS." Institute of Medicine Conference Summary, 1991.

Ezzyat, Youssef, et al. "Closed-Loop Stimulation of Temporal Cortex Rescues Functional Networks and Improves Memory." *Nature Communications* 9, no. 1 (February 2018): 365.

Faden, Ruth. "Ethical Issues in Government Sponsored Public Health Campaigns." *Health Education Quarterly* 14, no. 1 (1987): 27–37.

Faden, Ruth, and Tom L. Beauchamp. *A History and Theory of Informed Consent.* New York: Oxford University Press, 1986.

Falk, Emily B., and Danielle S. Bassett. "Brain and Social Networks: Fundamental Building Blocks of Human Experience." *Trends in Cognitive Science* 21, no. 9 (2017): 674–90.

Falk, Emily B., Elliot T. Berkman, Traci Mann, Brittany Harrison, and Matthew D. Lieberman. "Predicting Persuasion-Induced Behavior Change from the Brain." *Journal of Neuroscience* 30, no. 25 (June 2010): 8421–24.

Falk, Emily B., Matthew Brook O'Donnell, Steven Tompson, Richard Gonzalez, Sonya Dal Cin, Victor J. Strecher, Kenneth Michael Cummings, and Lawrence C. An. "Functional Brain Imaging Predicts Public Health Campaign Success." *Social Cognitive and Affective Neuroscience* 11, no. 2 (February 2016): 204–14.

Farahany, Nita, and James E. Coleman Jr. "Genetics, Neuroscience, and Criminal Responsibility." In *The Impact of the Behavioral Sciences on Criminal Law*, edited by Nita Farahany. New York: Oxford University Press, 2009: 183-240, 202.

Farahany, Nita A., et al. "The Ethics of Experimenting with Human Brain Tissue." *Nature* 556 (April 26, 2018): 429–32.

Fein, Rashi. "Toward Adequate Health Care: Why We Need National Health Insurance." *Dissent*, Winter 1988. http://dissent.syminic.com/article/toward-adequate-health-care-why-we-need-national-health-insurance.

Final Report of the Tuskegee Syphilis Study Ad Hoc Advisory Panel. April 28, 1973. http://www.research.usf.edu/dric/hrpp/foundations-course/docs/finalreport-tuskegeestudyadvisorypanel.pdf.

Finley, Allysia. "How HIV Became a Cancer Cure." *Wall Street Journal*, August 18, 2017. https://www.wsj.com/articles/how-hiv-became-a-cancer-cure-1503092082.

Fletcher, Joseph. *The Ethics of Genetic Control: Ending Reproductive Roulette.* New York: Anchor Press/Doubleday, 1974.

Food and Drug Administration. "FDA Approval Brings First Gene Therapy to the United States." August 30, 2017. https://www.fda.gov/NewsEvents/Newsroom/PressAnnouncements/ucm574058.htm.

———. "Kefauver-Harris Amendments Revolutionized Drug Development." Accessed September 14, 2018. https://www.fda.gov/ForConsumers/ConsumerUpdates/ucm 322856.htm.

———. "Notice of Initiation of Disqualification Proceeding and Opportunity to Explain." November 30, 2000. https://www.fda.gov/downloads/RegulatoryInforma tion/FOI/ElectronicReadingRoom/UCM144493.pdf.

Frakt, Austin. "Medical Mystery: Something Happened to U.S. Health Spending after 1980." *New York Times*, May 14, 2018. https://www.nytimes.com/2018/05/14/ upshot/medical-mystery-health-spending-1980.html.

"Front Matter." *Philosophy and Public Affairs* 1, no. 1 (Autumn 1971): 1–2.

Garnick, Marc B. "Filling in the Gaps." *Journal of the American Medical Association* 319, no. 20 (May 22/29, 2018): 2079–80.

Garrison, Jr., Louis P., Deborah Lubeck, Deepa Lalla, Virginia Paton, Amylou Dueck, Edith A. Perez. "Cost-Effectiveness Analysis of Trastuzumab in the Adjuvant Set- ting for Treatment of HER2-Positive Breast Cancer." *Cancer* 110, no.3 (August 1, 2007): 489-498.

Gawande, Atul. "The Cost Conundrum." *New Yorker*, June 1, 2009.

———. "Overkill." *New Yorker*, May 11, 2015.

———. "Why Doctors Hate Their Computers." *New Yorker*, November 12, 2018.

George, Robert P. *In Defense of Natural Law*. Oxford, UK: Oxford University Press, 2001.

Gibson, Daniel G., et al. "Creation of a Bacterial Cell Controlled by a Chemically Synthesized Genome." *Science* 329, no. 5987 (July 2010): 52–56.

Girgis, Sherif, Ryan T. Anderson, and Robert P. George. *What Is Marriage? Man and Woman: A Defense*. New York: Encounter Books, 2012.

———. "What Is Marriage?" *Harvard Journal of Law and Public Policy* 34, no. 1 (2010): 245–88.

Goel, Vindu. "Facebook Tinkers with Users' Emotions in News Feed Experi- ment, Stirring Outcry." *New York Times*, June 30, 2014. https://www.nytimes .com/2014/06/30/technology/facebook-tinkers-with-users-emotions-in-news-feed -experiment-stirring-outcry.html.

Gossman, Eva. *Good Beyond Evil: Ordinary People in Extraordinary Times*. London: Vallentine Mitchell, 2002.

Gostin, Lawrence O., Cori Vanchieri, and Andrew Pope, eds. *Ethical Considerations for Research Involving Prisoners*. Washington, DC: National Academies Press, 2007.

Gottlieb, Scott. "Remarks on FDA Approval of First Gene Therapy in the United States." August 30, 2017. https://www.fda.gov/NewsEvents/Speeches/ucm574113 .htm.

Grady, Denise. "Breakthrough Leukemia Treatment Backfires in a Rare Case." *New York Times*, October 1, 2018. https://www.nytimes.com/2018/10/01/health/ leukemia-immunotherapy-kymriah.html.

Greely, Henry T., Mildred K. Cho, Linda F. Hogle, and Debra M. Satz. "Thinking about the Human Neuron Mouse." *American Journal of Bioethics* 7, no. 5 (May 2007): 27–40.

Green, Dwight H. "Ethics Governing the Service of Prisoners as Subjects in Medical Experiments." *JAMA* 136, no. 7 (1948): 457–58.

Groopman, Jerome. "The Elusive Artificial Heart." *New York Review of Books*, November 22, 2018.

Guarino, Ben. "Researchers Clone the First Primates from Monkey Tissue Cells." *Washington Post*, January 24, 2018. https://www.washingtonpost.com/news/ speaking-of-science/wp/2018/01/24/researchers-clone-the-first-primates-from -monkey-tissue-cells/?utm_term=.fbe9f502d253.

Gutmann, Amy. "For and Against Equal Access to Health Care." *Milbank Memorial Fund Quarterly* 59, no. 4 (1984): 542–60.

Gutmann, Amy, and Jonathan D. Moreno. "Keep CRISPR Safe: Regulating a Genetic Revolution." *Foreign Affairs* (May/June 2018), 171–76.

Gutmann, Amy, and Dennis F. Thompson. *Democracy and Disagreement*. Cambridge, MA: Belknap Press, 1998.

———. *Why Deliberative Democracy?* Princeton, NJ: Princeton University Press, 2004.

Gutmann, Amy, and James W. Wagner. "Reflections on Democratic Deliberation in Bioethics." Special issue, *Hastings Center Report* (May/June 2017).

Halstead, John. "The Best Public Health Interventions of the 20th Century." *Giving What We Can*, April 25, 2015. https://www.givingwhatwecan.org/post/2015/04/ best-public-health-interventions-20th-century/.

Hardin, Garrett. "Lifeboat Ethics: The Case Against Helping the Poor." *Psychology Today*, September 1974.

Harkness, Jon M. "Nuremberg and the Issue of Wartime Experiments on US Prisoners: The Green Committee." *JAMA* 276, no. 20 (1996): 1672–75.

Hayden, Erika Check. "Privacy Protections: The Genome Hacker," *Nature* 497 (2016): 172–74.

Hayek, Friedrich A. *Law, Legislation and Liberty, Volume 2: The Mirage of Social Justice*. Chicago: University of Chicago Press, 1976.

———. *The Road to Serfdom*. New York: Routledge, 1944.

Hayes, Daniel F. Review of *False Hope: Bone Marrow Transplantation for Breast Cancer*, by Richard A. Rettig, Peter Jacobson, Cynthia M. Farquhar, and Wade M. Aubry. *New England Journal of Medicine* 357 (September 2007): 1059–60.

Hayes, Susan L., Sara R. Collins, David C. Radley, and Douglas McCarthy. "What's at Stake: State's Progress on Health Coverage and Access to Care, 2013–2016." Commonwealth Fund, December 14, 2017. https://www.commonwealthfund .org/publications/issue-briefs/2017/dec/whats-stake-states-progress-health -coverage-and-access-care-2013#/.

Healy, Edwin F. *Medical Ethics*. Chicago: Loyola University Press, 1956.

"Heart Surgeon Christiaan Barnard Dies." *Washington Post*, September 3, 2001. https://www.washingtonpost.com/archive/local/2001/09/03/heart-surgeon -christiaan-barnard-dies/82ab4aae-4854-462e-96b3-dbf042ecadf4/.

Helft, Miguel. "Googles Uses Searches to Track Flu's Spread." *New York Times*, November 12, 2008. https://www.nytimes.com/2008/11/12/technology/internet/12flu .html.

Heller, Jean. "Syphilis Victims in U.S. Study Went Untreated for 40 Years." *New York Times,* July 26, 1972, 1.

Hornblum, Allen M. *Acres of Skin: Human Experiments at Holmesburg Prison.* New York: Routledge, 1999.

———. "NYC's Forgotten Cancer Scandal." *New York Post,* December 28, 2013. https://nypost.com/2013/12/28/nycs-forgotten-cancer-scandal/.

Hudak, John, and Grace Wallack. "Ending the U.S. Government's War on Medical Marijuana Research." Center for Effective Governance at Brookings, June 2016. https://www.brookings.edu/wp-content/uploads/2016/06/Ending-the-US-governments-war-on-medical-marijuana-research.pdf.

Insel, Thomas. "Post by Former NIMH Director Thomas Insel: Mental Health Awareness Month: By the Numbers." May 5, 2015. https://www.nimh.nih.gov/about/directors/thomas-insel/blog/2015/mental-health-awareness-month-by-the-numbers.shtml.

International Bioethics Committee. "Report of the IBC on the Principle of Non-Discrimination and Non-Stigmatization." March 6, 2014. http://unesdoc.unesco.org/images/0022/002211/221196E.pdf.

International Registry in Organ Donation and Transplantation. "Final Numbers 2016." December 2017. http://www.irodat.org/img/database/pdf/IRODaT%20newletter%20Final%202016.pdf.

"It's Over, Debbie." *JAMA* 259, no. 2 (1988): 272.

Jacobson, Louis. "Does Emergency Care Account for Just 2 Percent of All Health Spending?" *Politifact,* October 28, 2013. https://www.politifact.com/truth-o-meter/statements/2013/oct/28/nick-gillespie/does-emergency-care-account-just-2-percent-all-hea/.

Johnson, Rebecca, Govin Persad, and Dominic Sisti. "The Tarasoff Rule: The Implications of Interstate Variation and Gaps in Professional Training." *Journal of the American Academy of Psychiatry and the Law Online* 42, no. 4 (2014): 469–77.

Jones, David S., Christine Grady, and Susan E. Lederer. "'Ethics and Clinical Research'—The 50th Anniversary of Beecher's Bombshell." *New England Journal of Medicine* 374, no. 24 (June 2016): 2393–98.

Jonsen, Albert R. *The Birth of Bioethics.* New York: Oxford University Press, 1998.

Jonsen, Albert R., and Stephen Toulmin. *The Abuse of Casuistry: A History of Moral Reasoning.* Berkeley: University of California Press, 1988.

Jouvenal, Justin. "To Find Alleged Golden State Killer, Investigators First Found His Great-Great-Great Grandparents." *Washington Post,* April 30, 2018. https://www.washingtonpost.com/local/public-safety/to-find-alleged-golden-state-killer-investigators-first-found-his-great-great-great-grandparents/2018/04/30/3c865fe7-dfcc-4a0e-b6b2-0bec548d501f_story.html.

Kahneman, Daniel. *Thinking, Fast and Slow.* New York: Farrar, Straus and Giroux, 2011.

Kandel, Eric R. *In Search of Memory: The Emergence of a New Science of Mind.* New York: W. W. Norton, 2006.

Kant, Immanuel. *Critique of Pure Reason* (1781). Cambridge: Cambridge University Press, 1999.

————. *Groundwork of the Metaphysics of Morals* (1785). Edited by Mary Gregor and Jens Timmermann. Cambridge: Cambridge University Press, 2012.

Karmali, Ruchir N., Natalie M. Jones, and Aaron D. Levine. "Tracking and Assessing the Rise of State-Funded Stem Cell Research." *Nature Biotechnology* 28, no. 12 (2010): 1246–48.

Kass, Leon R. "The End of Courtship." American Enterprise Institute, September 23, 2002. https://www.aei.org/publication/the-end-of-courtship/.

————. "Reflections on Public Bioethics: A View from the Trenches." *Kennedy Institute of Ethics Journal* 15, no. 3 (2005): 221–50.

Kass, Nancy. "An Ethics Framework for Public Health." *American Journal of Public Health* 91, no. 11 (2001): 1776–82.

Kateb, George. *Human Dignity.* Cambridge, MA: Harvard University Press, 2011.

Katz, Jay. "The Consent Principle of the Nuremberg Code: Its Significance Then and Now." In *The Nazi Doctors and the Nuremberg Code: Human Rights in Human Experimentation*, edited by George J. Annas and Michael A. Grodin, 228. New York: Oxford University Press, 1992.

————. *The Silent World of Doctor and Patient.* New York: Free Press, 1984.

Kelsey, Frances O. "Thalidomide Update: Regulatory Aspects." *Teratology* 38, no. 3 (1988): 221–26.

Kevles, Daniel J. "Why Is Medicine So Expensive." *New York Review of Books*, February 21, 2019. https://www.nybooks.com/articles/2019/02/21/why-is-medicine-so-expensive/.

Kevorkian, Jack. *Prescription: Medicide: The Goodness of Planned Death.* Amherst, NY: Prometheus Books, 1991.

Khazan, Olga. "Most Prisoners Are Mentally Ill." *Atlantic*, April 7, 2015. https://www.theatlantic.com/health/archive/2015/04/more-than-half-of-prisoners-are-mentally-ill/389682/.

Klein, Rich, and Jennifer Parker. "Politics of Stem Cell Debate in Flux." June 20, 2007. https://abcnews.go.com/Politics/story?id=3297955&page=1.

Kolata, Gina B. "Dialysis after Nearly a Decade." *Science* 208, no. 4443 (May 1980): 473–76.

Kopp, Vincent J. "Henry Knowles Beecher and the Development of Informed Consent in Anesthesia Research." *Anesthesiology* 90, no. 6 (1999): 1756–65.

Krugman, Saul. "The Willowbrook Hepatitis Studies Revisited: Ethical Aspects." *Reviews of Infectious Diseases* 8, no. 1 (1986): 157–62.

Lander, Eric S. "The Heroes of CRISPR." *Cell* 164 (2016): 24–25.

Lehmann, Evan. "Conservatives Lose Faith in Science over Last 40 Years." *Scientific American*, March 30, 2012. https://www.scientificamerican.com/article/conservatives-lose-faith-in-science-over-last-40-years/.

Lepore, Jill. "The Politics of Death." *New Yorker*, November 30, 2009. https://www.newyorker.com/magazine/2009/11/30/the-politics-of-death.

Letters to the Editor. *JAMA* 259, no. 14 (1988): 2094–95.

Levy, David T., Zhe Yuan, Yuying Luo, and Darren Mays. "Seven Years of Progress in Tobacco Control: An Evaluation of the Effect of Nations Meeting the Highest Level MPOWER Measures between 2007 and 2014." *Tobacco Control* 27, no. 1 (2018): 50–57.

Libertarian Party. 2018 Platform. Accessed September 14, 2018. https://www.lp.org/platform/.

Locke, John. *Two Treatises of Government (1690)*. Edited by Peter Laslett. Cambridge: Cambridge University Press, 1988.

Lombardo, Paul, ed. *A Century of Eugenics in America: From the Indiana Experiment to the Human Genome Era*. Bloomington: Indiana University Press, 2011.

Macedo, Stephen. *Just Married: Same-Sex Couples, Monogamy & the Future of Marriage*. Princeton, NJ: Princeton University Press, 2015.

Macklin, Ruth. "Dignity Is a Useless Concept: It Means No More Than Respect for Persons or Their Autonomy." *British Medical Journal* 327, no. 7429 (December 2003): 1419–20.

Mahoney, Julia D. "Altruism, Markets, and Organ Procurement." *Law and Contemporary Problems* 72 (2009): 17–36.

Maley, Terry. *Democracy & the Political in Max Weber's Thought*. Toronto: University of Toronto Press, 2011.

Masters, Rebecca, Elspeth Anwar, Brendan Collins, Richard Cookson, and Simon Capewell. "Return on Investment of Public Health Interventions: A Systematic Review." *Journal of Epidemiology and Community Health* 71, no. 8 (August 2017): 827–34.

Matjasko, Jennifer L., John H. Cawley, Madeleine M. Baker-Goering, and Dvaid V. Yokum. "Applying Behavioral Economics to Public Health Policy: Illustrative Examples and Promising Directions." *American Journal of Preventive Medicine* 50, no. 5 Suppl 1 (May 2016): S13–19.

Maude, Shannon L., Noelle V. Frey, Pamela A. Shaw, Richard Aplenc, David M. Barrett, Nancy J. Bunin, Anne Chew, Vanessa E. Gonzalez, Zhaohui Zheng, Simon F. Lacey, Yolanda D. Mahnke, Jan Joseph Melenhorst, Susan R. Rheingold, Angela Shen, David Teachey, Bruce L. Levine, Carl H. June, David L. Porter, and Stephan A. Grupp. "Chimeric Antigen Receptor T Cells for Sustained Remissions in Leukemia." *New England Journal of Medicine* 371 (October 2014): 1507–17.

Maynard, Brittany. "My Right to Death with Dignity at 29." CNN, November 2, 2014. http://www.cnn.com/2014/10/07/opinion/maynard-assisted-suicide-cancer-dignity/index.html.

McCaffrey, James P. "Hospital Accused on Cancer Study; Live Cells Given to Patients without Their Consent, Director Tells Court; Allegation Is Denied; Chronic Disease Institution Defends Action—Value of Tests Is Praised." *New York Times*, January 21, 1964, 31, 51.

McCarthy, Meghan. "Seniors Love Their Medicare (Advantage)." *Morning Consult*, March 30, 2015. https://morningconsult.com/2015/03/30/seniors-love-their-medicare-advantage/.

McCrystal, Laura. "Pa. Supreme Court Upholds Philadelphia Soda Tax." July 18, 2018. http://www2.philly.com/philly/news/soda-tax-philadelphia-supreme-court-pennsylvania-20180718.html.

McElhinney, Thomas K., and Edmund D. Pellegrino. "The Institute on Human Values in Medicine: Its Role and Influence in the Conception and Evolution of Bio-ethics." *Theoretical Medicine and Bioethics* 22, no. 4 (August 2001): 291–317.

McFadden, Robert D. "Frances Oldham Kelsey, Who Saved U.S. Babies from Tha-lidomide, Dies at 101." *New York Times*, August 7, 2015. https://www.nytimes .com/2015/08/08/science/frances-oldham-kelsey-fda-doctor-who-exposed-danger -of-thalidomide-dies-at-101.html.

McKellar, Shelley. *Artificial Hearts: The Allure and Ambivalence of a Controversial Medical Technology.* Baltimore: Johns Hopkins University Press, 2018.

Merz, Jon F., Catherine A. Jackson, and Jacob Alex Klerman. "A Review of Abor-tion Policy: Legality, Medicaid Funding, and Parental Involvement, 1967–1994." *Women's Rights Law Report* 17, no. 1 (Winter 1995): 1–61.

Miller, Richard B. *Casuistry and Modern Ethics: A Poetics of Practical Reasoning.* Chi-cago: University of Chicago Press, 1996.

Moreno, Jonathan D. "The First Scientist to 'Play God' Was Not Craig Venter." *Science Progress*, May 25, 2010. https://scienceprogress.org/2010/05/synbio-ethics/.

———. "How a Zika Virus Breakthrough Vindicates Stem Cell Research." *Huff-Post*, March 16, 2017. https://www.huffingtonpost.com/jonathan-d-moreno/how -a-zika-virus-breakthr_b_9472846.html.

———. "Why We Need to Be More Accepting of 'Humanized' Lab Animals." *Atlan-tic*, October 2011. https://www.theatlantic.com/health/archive/2011/10/why-we -need-to-be-more-accepting-of-humanized-lab-animals/246071/.

Moreno, Jonathan D., Ulf Schmidt, and Steve Joffe. "The Nuremberg Code 70 Years Later." *JAMA* 318, no. 9 (2017): 795–96.

National Academies of Sciences, Engineering, and Medicine. *The Health Effects of Cannabis and Cannabinoids: The Current State of Evidence and Recommendations for Research.* Washington, DC: National Academies Press, 2017.

———. *Human Genome Editing: Science, Ethics, and Governance.* Washington, DC: National Academies Press, 2017.

———. *Mitochondrial Replacement Techniques: Ethical, Social, and Policy Consider-ations.* Washington, DC: National Academies Press, 2016.

The National Commission for the Protection of Human Subjects of Biomedical and Behavioral Research. *The Belmont Report: Ethics Principles and Guidelines for the Protection of Human Subjects of Research.* Washington, DC, 1979. https://www .hhs.gov/ohrp/regulations-and-policy/belmont-report/read-the-belmont-report/ index.html.

National Research Council and Institute of Medicine of the National Academies. *Guidelines for Human Embryonic Stem Cell Research.* Washington, DC: National Academies Press, 2005.

Novack, Dennis H., Robin Plumer, Raymond L. Smith, Herbert Ochitill, Gary R. Morrow, and John M. Bennett. "Changes in Physicians' Attitudes toward Telling the Cancer Patient." *JAMA* 241, no. 9 (March 1979): 897–900.

Nozick, Robert. *Anarchy, State, and Utopia.* New York: Basic Books, 1974.

Nuffield Council on Bioethics. *The Collection, Linking and Use of Data in Biomedical Research and Health Care: Ethical Issues.* February 2015. http://nuffieldbioethics .org/wp-content/uploads/Biological_and_health_data_web.pdf.

The Nuremberg Code. Accessed September 14, 2018. https://history.nih.gov/research/downloads/nuremberg.pdf.

Nurkin, Steven. "Symptoms of Colon Cancer in Women." *RoswellPark.org*, March 23, 2018. https://www.roswellpark.org/cancertalk/201803/symptoms-colon-cancer-women.

Obama, Barack. Executive Order 13505. Accessed September 14, 2018. https://www.gpo.gov/fdsys/pkg/DCPD-200900136/content-detail.html;https://www.gpo.gov/fdsys/pkg/FR-2009-03-11/pdf/E9-5441.pdf.

O'Callaghan, Martine. "Autism: A Mother's Story." *Vaccines Today*, June 22, 2012. https://www.vaccinestoday.eu/stories/autism-a-mothers-story/.

Oken, Donald. "What to Tell Cancer Patients: A Study of Medical Attitudes." *JAMA* 175, no. 13 (1961): 1120–28.

Organ Donation and Transplantation Activities, 2015 Report. Accessed September 14, 2018. http://www.transplant-observatory.org/organ-donation-transplantation-activities-2015-report-2/.

Packard, Vance. *The Hidden Persuaders*, reissue ed. New York: IG, 2007.

Papanicolas, Irene, Liana R. Woskie, and Ashish K. Jha. "Health Care Spending in the United States and Other High-Income Countries." *JAMA* 319, no. 10 (March 2018): 1024–39.

Pear, Robert. "New Medicare Rule Authorizes 'End-of-Life Consultations.'" *New York Times*, October 31, 2015. https://www.nytimes.com/2015/10/31/us/new-medicare-rule-authorizes-end-of-life-consultations.html.

———. "'Short Term' Health Insurance? Up to 3 Years under New Trump Policy." *New York Times*, August 1, 2018. https://www.nytimes.com/2018/08/01/us/politics/trump-short-term-health-insurance.html.

Pew Research Center. "The American Middle Class Is Losing Ground." December 2015.

———. "Public Support for 'Single Payer' Health Coverage Grows, Driven by Democrats." July 2017.

Please Let Me Die, produced by Dax Cowert and Robert White (1974), DVD.

Porter, David L., Bruce L. Levine, Michael Kalos, Adam Bagg, and Carl H. June. "Chimeric Antigen Receptor-Modified T Cells in Chronic Lymphoid Leukemia." *New England Journal of Medicine* 365, no. 8 (August 2011): 725–33.

Presidential Commission for the Study of Bioethical Issues. *Bioethics for Every Generation: Deliberation and Education in Health, Science and Technology*. Washington, DC, May 2016. https://bioethicsarchive.georgetown.edu/pcsbi/sites/default/files/PCSBI_Bioethics-Deliberation_0.pdf.

———. *Ethically Impossible: STD Research in Guatemala from 1946 to 1948*. Washington, DC, 2011. https://bioethicsarchive.georgetown.edu/pcsbi/sites/default/files/Ethically%20Impossible%20(with%20linked%20historical%20documents)%202.7.13.pdf.

———. *Gray Matters: Integrative Approaches for Neuroscience, Ethics, and Society, Volume 1*. Washington, DC, 2014. http://www.bioethics.gov/sites/default/files/Gray%20Matters%20Vol%201.pdf.

———. *Gray Matters: Integrative Approaches for Neuroscience, Ethics, and Society, Volume 2.* Washington, DC, 2015. https://bioethicsarchive.georgetown.edu/pcsbi/sites/default/files/GrayMatter_V2_508.pdf.

———. *New Directions: The Ethics of Synthetic Biology and Emerging Technologies.* Washington, DC, 2010. https://bioethicsarchive.georgetown.edu/pcsbi/sites/default/files/PCSBI-Synthetic-Biology-Report-12.16.10_0.pdf.

———. *Safeguarding Children: Pediatric Medical Countermeasure Research.* Washington, DC, 2013. https://bioethicsarchive.georgetown.edu/pcsbi/sites/default/files/PCSBI_Pediatric-MCM508.pdf.

President's Commission for the Study of Ethical Problems in Medicine and Biomedical and Behavioral Research. *Deciding to Forego Life-Sustaining Treatment.* Washington, DC, 1983.

———. *Securing Access to Health Care.* Washington, DC, 1983.

"Prison Malaria: Convicts Expose Themselves to Disease so Doctors Can Study It." *Life Magazine,* June 4, 1945, 43–46.

"Privacy Best Practices for Consumer Genetic Testing Services." https://fpf.org/wp-content/uploads/2018/07/Privacy-Best-Practices-for-Consumer-Genetic-Testing-Services-FINAL.pdf, accessed 9/14/2018.

Quigley, Muireann. "Nudging for Health: On Public Policy and Designing Choice Architecture." *Medical Law Review* 21, no. 4 (2013): 588–621.

Quill, Timothy E. "Death and Dignity: A Case of Individualized Decision Making." *New England Journal of Medicine* 324 (1991): 691–94.

———. *Death and Dignity: Making Choices and Taking Charge.* New York: W. W. Norton, 1994.

Quill, Timothy E., Robert M. Arnold, and Stuart J. Youngner. "Physician-Assisted Suicide: Finding a Path Forward in a Changing Legal Environment." *Annals of Internal Medicine* 167, no. 8 (October 2017): 597–98.

Rabkin, Mitchell T., Gerald Gillerman, and Nancy R. Rice. "Orders Not to Resuscitate." *New England Journal of Medicine* 295 (August 1976): 364–66.

Raine, Adrian. *The Anatomy of Violence: The Biological Roots of Crime.* New York: Random House, 2013.

Ramsey, Paul. *Fabricated Man: The Ethics of Genetic Control.* New Haven, CT: Yale University Press, 1970.

Rawls, John. *A Theory of Justice: Revised Edition.* Cambridge: Belknap Press, 1999.

Reardon, Sarah. "'Three-Parent Baby' Claim Raises Hope—and Ethical Concerns." *Nature,* September 29, 2016. https://www.nature.com/news/three-parent-baby-claim-raises-hopes-and-ethical-concerns-1.20698.

Regalado, Antonio. "23andMe Sells Data for Drug Search." *MIT Technology Review,* June 21, 2016. https://www.technologyreview.com/s/601506/23andme-sells-data-for-drug-search/.

Rettig, Richard A. "Origins of the Medicare Kidney Disease Entitlement: The Social Security Amendments of 1972." In *Biomedical Politics,* edited by K. E. Hanna. Washington, DC: National Academy Press, 1991.

———. "The Policy Debate on End-Stage Renal Disease," *Law and Contemporary*

Problems 40 (1976). Reprinted in *Ethics & Politics: Cases and Comments,* 1st ed., edited by A. Gutmann and D. Thompson. Chicago: Nelson-Hall, 1984.

Reverby, Susan M. "'Normal Exposure' and Inoculation Syphilis: A PHS 'Tuskegee' Doctor in Guatemala, 1946–48." *Journal of Policy History* 23 (2011): 6–28.

———. "Normal Exposure" and Inoculation Syphilis: PHS "Tuskegee." Doctors in Guatemala, 1946–48 and at Sing Sing Prison, Ossining, New York, 1953–54. Paper presented at the annual meeting of the American Association for the History of Medicine, Mayo Clinic, Rochester, MN, May 2, 2010.

Robinson, Walter M., and Brandon T. Unruh. "The Hepatitis Experiments at the Willowbrook State School." In *The Oxford Textbook of Clinical Research Ethics,* edited by Ezekiel J. Emanuel, Christine C. Grady, Robert A. Crouch, Reidar K. Lie, Franklin G. Miller, and David D. Wendler. New York: Oxford University Press, 2008.

Rosenthal, Elizabeth. "Nine Rights Every Patient Should Demand." *New York Times,* April 27, 2018. https://www.nytimes.com/2018/04/27/opinion/sunday/patients -rights-hospitals-health-care.html.

Rothman, David J. *Strangers at the Bedside: A History of How Law and Bioethics Transformed Medical Decision Making.* New York: Basic Books, 1991.

Rotterdam School of Management, Erasmus University. RSM Discovery (blog). *Identifying Strong Brands in the Brain.* June 8, 2018. https://discovery.rsm.nl/articles/ detail/348-strong-brands-can-be-identified-in-the-brain/.

Sacks, Oliver. *Awakenings.* Reprint ed. New York: Vintage, 1999.

———. *Musicophilia: Tales of Music and the Brain.* New York: Knopf, 2007.

Safier, Paul. "Rationing the Public: The Oregon Health Plan." In *Ethics & Politics: Cases and Comments.* 4th ed. Edited by A. Gutmann and D. Thompson. Chicago: Nelson-Hall, 2006.

Sandel, Michael. *What Money Can't Buy: The Moral Limits of Markets.* New York: Farrar, Straus, and Giroux, 2013.

Sanger-Katz, Margot, and Quoctrung Bui. "The Impact of Obamacare in Four Maps." *New York Times,* October 31, 2016. https://www.nytimes.com/interactive/2016/10/ 31/upshot/up-uninsured-2016.html.

Savitt, Todd. "The Use of Blacks for Medical Experimentation and Demonstration in the Old South." *Journal of Southern History* 48, no. 3 (1982): 331–48.

Scheufele, Dietram A., Michael A. Xenos, Emily L. Howell, Kathleen M. Rose, Dominique Brossard, and Bruce W. Hardy. "U.S. Attitudes on Human Genome Editing." *Science* 357, no. 6351 (August 2017): 553–54.

Scull, Andrew. *Madness in Civilization: A Cultural History of Insanity, from the Bible to Freud, from the Madhouse to Modern Medicine.* Kindle ed. Princeton, NJ: Princeton University Press, 2015.

Segal, Andrea G., Rosemary Frasso, and Dominic A. Sisti. "County Jail or Psychiatric Hospital? Ethical Challenges in Correctional Mental Health Care." *Qualitative Health Research* 28, no. 6 (2018): 963–76.

Sen, Amartya. *Commodities and Capabilities.* New York: Oxford University Press, 1999.

———. "Universal Health Care: The Affordable Dream." *Harvard Public Health*

Review 4 (2015). http://harvardpublichealthreview.org/universal-health-care-the -affordable-dream/.

Shamblott, Michael J., Joyce Axelman, S. P. Wang, Elizabeth M. Bugg, John W. Littlefield, Peter J. Donovan, Paul D. Blumenthal, George R. Huggins, and John D. Gearhart. "Derivation of Pluripotent Stem Cells from Cultured Human Primordial Germ Cells." *PNAS* 95, no. 23 (November 1998): 13726–31

Sherman, Ted. "N.J. Gay Couple Fight for Custody of Twin 5-Year-Old Girls." December 20, 2011. https://www.nj.com/news/index.ssf/2011/12/nj_gay_couple_ fight_for_custod.html.

Singer, Natasha. "Making Ads That Whisper to the Brain." *New York Times*, November 13, 2010. https://www.nytimes.com/2010/11/14/business/14stream.html.

Singer, Peter. *Animal Liberation*. New York: HarperCollins, 1975.

Sisti, Dominic A., Andrea G. Segal, and Ezekiel J. Emanuel. "Improving Long-Term Psychiatric Care: Bring Back the Asylum." *JAMA* 313, no. 3 (2015): 243–44.

Sisti, Dominic A., Elizabeth A. Sinclair, and Steven S. Sharfstein. "Bedless Psychiatry—Rebuilding Behavioral Health Service Capacity." *JAMA Psychiatry* 75, no. 5 (2018): 417–18.

Skloot, Rebecca. *The Immortal Life of Henrietta Lacks*. New York: Broadway Books, 2011.

Span, Paula. "A Quiet End to the 'Death Panels' Debate." *New York Times*, November 24, 2015. https://www.nytimes.com/2015/11/24/health/end-of-death-panels -myth-brings-new-end-of-life-challenges.html.

Starr, Paul. *The Social Transformation of American Medicine: The Rise of a Sovereign Profession and the Making of a Vast Industry*. New York: Basic Books, 1982.

"Statement from Michael R. Bloomberg on Philadelphia's Tax on Sugar Sweetened Beverages." June 16, 2016. https://www.mikebloomberg.com/news/statement -from-michael-r-bloomberg-on-philadelphias-tax-on-sugar-sweetened-beverages/.

Stevens, Rosemary. "Health Care in the Early 1960s." *Health Care Financing Review* 18, no. 2 (1996): 11–22.

Stolberg, Sheryl Gay. "Obama Is Leaving Some Stem Cell Issues to Congress." *New York Times*, March 8, 2009. https://www.nytimes.com/2009/03/09/us/ politics/09stem.html.

Sulmasy, Daniel. "Chapter 18: Dignity and Bioethics: History, Theory, and Selected Applications." In *Human Dignity and Bioethics: Essays Commissioned by the Presidents' Council on Bioethics*. Washington, DC, March 2008. https://bioethicsarchive .georgetown.edu/pcbe/reports/human_dignity/chapter18.html.

———. "Health Care Justice and Hospice Care." Supplement, *Hastings Center Report* 33, no. 2 (2003): S14–15. https://www.growthhouse.org/nhwg/sulmasy_ supplement.htm.

Sulmasy, Daniel P., and Edmund D. Pellegrino. "The Rule of Double Effect: Clearing Up the Double Talk." *Archives of Internal Medicine* 159, no. 6 (March 1999): 545–50.

Takahashi, Kazutoshi, Koji Tanabe, Mari Ohnuki, Megumi Narita, Tomoko Ichisaka, Kiichiro Tomoda, and Shinya Yamanaka. "Induction of Pluripotent Stem

Cells from Adult Human Fibroblasts by Defined Factors." *Cell* 131, no. 5 (November 2007): 861–72.

Tandy-Connor, Stephany, Jenna Guiltinan, Kate Krempely, Holly LaDuca, Patrick Reineke, Stephanie Gutierrez, Phillip Gray, and Brigette Tippin Davis. "False-Positive Results Released by Direct-to-Consumer Genetics Tests Highlight the Importance of Clinical Confirmation Testing for Appropriate Patient Care." *Genetics in Medicine* (2018).

Tennison, Michael N., and Amanda C. Pustilnik. "'And If Your Friends Jumped Off a Bridge, Would You Do It Too?' How Developmental Neuroscience Can Inform Legal Regimes Governing Adolescents." *Indiana Health Law Review* 12, no. 2 (2015): 534–85.

Thaler, Richard. "Nudge, Not Sludge." *Science* 361, no. 6401 (2018): 431.

Thaler, Richard H., and Cass R. Sunstein. *Nudge: Improving Decisions about Health, Wealth, and Happiness.* Rev. ed. New York: Penguin Books, 2009.

Thomas, Katie. "Insurers Battle Families over Costly Drug for Fatal Disease." *New York Times,* June 22, 2017. https://www.nytimes.com/2017/06/22/health/duchenne-muscular-dystrophy-drug-exondys-51.html.

Thomas, Lewis. "The Technology of Medicine." *New England Journal of Medicine* 285 (1971): 1366–68.

Thompson, Dennis F. "The Problem of Many Hands." *American Political Science Review* 74, no. 4 (1980): 905–16.

Thomson, James A., Joseph Itskovitz-Eldor, Sander S. Shapiro, Michelle A. Waknitz, Jennifer J. Swiergiel, Vivienne S. Marshall, and Jeffrey M. Jones. "Embryonic Stem Cell Lines Derived from Human Blastocysts." *Science* 282, no. 5391 (November 1998): 1145–47.

Thomson, Judith Jarvis. "A Defense of Abortion." *Philosophy and Public Affairs* 1, no. 1 (1971): 47–66.

Toffler, Alvin. *Future Shock.* New York: Bantam, 1984.

Trials of War Criminals Before the Nuernberg Military Tribunals, Vol. 1. Washington, DC: U.S. Government Printing Office, 1949.

UCR. "Poor Ben Casey! Dr. Maggie's Switching Roles from That of Anesthesiologist." *Desert Sun* 36, no. 268 (June 14, 1963), 14.

"UK's Independent Expert Panel Recommends 'Cautious Adoption' of Mitochondrial Donation in Treatment." October 10, 2017. https://www.hfea.gov.uk/about-us/news-and-press-releases/2016-news-and-press-releases/uks-independent-expert-panel-recommends-cautious-adoption-of-mitochondrial-donation-in-treatment/.

Wagner, Caroline S. *The New Invisible College.* Washington, D.C.: Brookings Institution Press, 2008.

Wakefield, A. J., Simon H. Murch, Andrew Anthony, John Linnell, D. M. Casson, Mohsin Malik, Mark Berelowitz, A. P. Dhillon, M. A. Thomson, P. Harvey, Alan Valentine, Susan Davies, and John Walker-Smith. "RETRACTED: Ileal-Lymphoid-Nodular Hyperplasia, Non-Specific Colitis, and Pervasive Developmental Disorder in Children." *Lancet* 351, no. 9103 (February 1998): 637–41.

Waldron, Jeremy. "It's All for Your Own Good." *New York Review of Books,* October 9, 2014.

Waxman, Henry, Bill Corr, Kristi Martin, and Sophia Duong. "Getting to the Root of High Prescription Drug Prices: Drivers and Potential Solutions." CommonwealthFund.org, July 10, 2017, https://www.commonwealth fund.org/publications/fund-reports/2017/jul/getting-root-high-prescription -drug-prices-drivers-and-potential.

Weiss, Rick. "Clinton Forbids Funding of Human Clone Studies." *Washington Post*, March 5, 1997. https://www.washingtonpost.com/archive/politics/1997/03/05/ clinton-forbids-funding-of-human-clone-studies/3b2f831f-f23e-4457-8611 -6c9bda0b8ebf/.

Wertheimer, Roger. "Understanding the Abortion Argument." *Philosophy and Public Affairs* 1, no. 1 (1971): 67–95.

Will, George F. "Affirming a Right to Die with Dignity." *Washington Post*, August 25, 2015. https://www.washingtonpost.com/opinions/distinctions-in-end-of-life -decisions/2015/08/28/b34b8f6a-4ce7-11e5-902f-39e9219e574b_story.html.

Williams, Roger. "The Nazis and Thalidomide: The Worst Drug Scandal of All Time." *Newsweek*, September 10, 2012.

Wilson, Robin Fretwell. "The Death of Jesse Gelsinger: New Evidence of the Influence of Money and Prestige in Human Research." *American Journal of Law and Medicine* 36 (2010): 295–325.

Yu, Junying, Maxim A. Vodyanik, Kim Smuga-Otto, Jessica Antosiewicz-Bourget, Jennifer L. Frane, Shulan Tian, Jeff Nie, Gudrun A. Jonsdottir, Victor Ruotti, Ron Stewart, Igor I. Slukvin, and James A. Thomson. "Induced Pluripotent Stem Cell Lines Derived from Human Somatic Cells." *Science* 318, no. 5858 (December 2007): 1917–20.

Zimmer, Carl. *She Has Her Mother's Laugh: The Powers, Perversions, and Potential of Heredity.* New York: Dutton, 2018.

INDEX

Page numbers followed by *n* refer to notes.